THE ORGAN HARVESTERS

Other novels by Bette Golden Lamb

The Organ Harvesters-Book II

Novels by Bette Golden Lamb & J. J. Lamb

Sisters in Silence
Heir Today...
The Killing Vote
(Gina Mazzio, RN Medical Thriller Series)
Bone Dry
Sin & Bone
Bone Pit
Bone of Contention
Bone Dust
Bone Crack

THE ORGAN HARVESTERS

by

Bette Golden Lamb

Two Black Sheep Productions
Novato, California

www.bettelamb.com

Originally published in soft cover and electronically by Farther Books, an imprint of Assent Publishing.

ISBN-13: 978-0-9984643-0-5
ISBN-10: 0-9984643-0-9

Dedication

For J. J.:
My partner, my lover, my forever best friend.

Chapter 1

Dr. Zoe Hidalga jumped back as a sudden splat of green slime blossomed on her plastin face shield. A mental image of her eyes drenched in caustic acid filled her brain. She shivered and quickly looked around to see if any of the other doctors had noticed her clumsiness, but they were all in their final thirty minutes of a nine-hour shift. No time or interest to observe her problem. Quotas had to be met.

The splash of gore had come from a diseased gallbladder she'd just peeled away from a healthy liver. Her heart was still crashing against her chest as she leaned over to study the slippery brown mass before lowering it into a four-liter, see-through container labeled *Organ Acceptable*.

She tossed the useless gallbladder sac onto a waste conveyor and watched the moving belt snake its way through the room as it carried other organic disposable products to the disintegration chamber. Disgusted with her clumsiness, she cleaned away the residue of bile from her mask and tossed it on the marble dissection table.

A blast of static from a loudspeaker filled the maze of cubicles, followed by the sound of strident voices announcing, "*Terrorists will not win. We need Corporit protection. We need Corporit justice.*"

Palpable unease rippled across the room. Zoe took a deep breath and tried to harness the noise by reconfiguring it into the wild, dissonant horns of a Clifford overture. But it was what it was: a warning that their daily ration of Corporit National Council propaganda was about to begin.

Elections were ten months away and the chorus of shouting voices promised citizen protection from the murderous terrorists and the violence of the homeless tribes. They also promised new medicine to cure the rampant spread of disease. Zoe cringed as the voices droned on. They talked about terrorists breaking into apartments, hurting and killing people—fearful everyday events that held her and everyone else's attention like fingers squeezing her neck.

Before she could pick up the next bag of human viscera, the production line slowed to a halt. She glanced at the clock to assure her that it was actually time to quit and not just an equipment malfunction.

1630.

It was over. Only sheer willpower had gotten her through the last two hours of the shift.

She stepped away from her stool, staggered, and reached out for the sides of her cubicle to keep from falling. She was growing weaker.

Weaker every day.

It took longer than usual to complete her production report and enter it into the computer. She studied her output numbers, then swallowed hard when she realized it was the third day in a row she hadn't met the daily work quota.

Part of her didn't care; she hated the job and the cramped space where she was trapped like a rat. But her position as an organ evacuator left her hanging on to the lowest rung on the Corporit harvesting ladder. There was no place left to work and remain part of the Corporit medical system—at least not with her limited medical orientation. Zoe had to succeed or become homeless.

By the time she completed her report, she was the last of the dozen Viscer-Surg doctors to leave the lab. At least no one would witness the physical effort it took for her to make her way out of the complex.

* * *

The stench of organ preservative lingered in Zoe's nostrils as she stepped into the street- level transit station. It was crowded not only with passengers, but with squadrons of uniformed military personnel, weapons armed and ready. Dark bulletproof visors shielded their watchful eyes; tense body language exposed their readiness to use their guns and tasers for any actual or presumed threat.

Zoe automatically tugged at the identification tag that hung loosely around her neck to make sure she hadn't forgotten it and its electronic identifier.

Breathing became increasingly difficult for Zoe as she stood outside her workplace. The protective dome, along with the air scrubbers and increased oxygen pressure inside the buildings, remained the only efficient shield against the polluted air that smothered ambient oxygen. She pulled a traveling oxygen container from her backpack and tugged on the nasal tube. When the air started to flow, her panic ebbed. She hated wearing the gear and could breathe without it if respiratory diseases didn't immediately gain a foothold and start her on a downward spiral of pulmonary destruction.

Craning her neck to search for the electro-magno express pod, she heard a child whine, "Mommy, that woman stinks." The child pointed at Zoe and held his nose while he yanked at his mother's hand, tugging her in the opposite direction. Other commuters took the boy's lead and edged away from Zoe, mumbling similar complaints.

"She's dirty," the child said aloud.

Zoe's face grew hot, but she refused to look at any one person. To cover her embarrassment, she stared at the hazy sky through the station's amber-tinted roof, but it only made things worse. She was just as trapped in here as she was in the laboratory.

Everyone was trapped in one way or another. Trapped on a dying planet.

Was there a time when they didn't have to live under the massive domes where scrubbed air was piped in and rising temperatures were neutralized?

Zoe remembered when she had lived in a real house with her parents. Sometimes a flash of memory gave her a fleeting view of a zoo, meadows, water ponds, even the splendor of a visit to a grove of giant redwoods. But many of those memories were turning into shadowy glimpses that were almost gone, like the glaciers and the vast forests with their oxygen-producing trees.

Now everything on the globe was dead or dying from the drought, the unrelenting heat, and the scourge of the fatal Viral Mal-Absorption Syndrome, a quirky mutation of the AIDS virus.

Deadly environment. Deadly disease.

Soon no one would survive inside or outside the domes, and when all the remaining trees were gone, life on Earth would end.

Zoe sighed, wasting the air left in her chest.

If only she and her daughter could run away to live in the Noncorp areas outside of San Francorp. At least she would be free. But everyday Corporit communications made the area sound not only desperate but disorganized. Out there were hostiles, the unemployed, and the unknown.

Would the bleak landscape and exposure to the elements be better than being trapped inside this covered city?

The thought of running away was an easy daydream until her chest tightened at the thought of breathing the polluted outside air. Could she put her little girl through that?

When her pod arrived, she sat down and held onto the seat's armrest, jittering with vibrations as the anti-grav vehicle sped between the city's towering structures.

In the past two years, a web-like array of interconnecting passageways had been completed, joining all the city's buildings. San Francorp's employees were now housed in tiny, expensive urban compounds. Suburban homes eroded outside of the domes: deserted, disintegrating, ghostly skeletons that dotted the dying landscape.

She yearned for signs of color, plant life, living creatures. Her hunger for the outdoors never seemed to be satisfied. Looking through the windows, she captured a fleeting glance of a bleak landscape. And even that was almost obliterated with the spread of uniform concrete-gray edifices, distinguished only by the mundane names emblazoned on each building: Corporit Department Store, Corporit Museum, Corporit Pharmaceuticals.

She had been in the pod for fifteen minutes when a sign

reading *Corporit Singles Complex #7* loomed like an eerie apparition floating from the skyline.

She pulled herself up and leaned her head against a pole until they pulled into the bowels of the building. She sighed and stepped out of the pod; the organ preservative essence preceded and followed her.

Zoe held her identification card up to the scanner and pressed her second and third fingertips against the DNA sensor to signal the vaculift. Once inside the lift, she braced herself against the wall for support, counting silently as the digital readout blinked each level.

At 19, the car eased to a stop. "This is your floor, Doctor Hidalga."

Zoe grimaced at the metallic, computer-generated voice and made her way down the long, cement corridor to her apartment.

* * *

Asher Wind Storm sat on an arid hilltop overlooking a landscape of desolation. Not a hint of animal, insect, or plant life existed in the leached soil that lifted and scattered in a final surrender to each wisp of wind. In the center of a large circle formed by his closest companions, he reached out and gently sifted through the lifeless dirt with probing fingers—the earth sucked the moisture from his calloused hands like a thirsty beast. He gathered the particles into tiny mounds. A sudden wind gust swallowed each pile, morphing the grains into a dust devil that swelled, lifted up, and reached out to the heavens. The swirl hung, suspended like a black angry cloud before it changed into a hovering apparition of an amber eye that stared through the thick, suffocating particles surrounding the planet.

The cloud drifted. It traveled farther and farther across the sterile landscape, tossing the dead soil that had not felt the softness of moisture or the swelling of growth for a long, hard decade.

When the eye returned to focus on the Medicine Wheel, a single tear fell from the sky and landed in the center of the circle.

Storm watched the tear settle at his feet. He planted three seeds in that single spot of moisture.

"Together, we must search through the vastness of the cosmos until we reach into the spheres of endless time. Once there, we will gather the embryos of universal life and bring them back to heal our Mother."

"Thrive." He held his hands over the seeds.

"We are at peace with all our brothers and sisters. One with all the spirits of our Earth. One with the oceans, rivers, rocks, soil, sky, plants, animals.

"We are them as they are us.

"We are all one."

Chapter 2

Cable Car Conglomerate
Corporit Singles Complex #7

Today, Zoe's cramped apartment seemed even smaller than usual. She moved past the drab, brown, two-seater sofa and went to the only window, which looked down onto a deserted gray street. She couldn't get away from the stench of her used, dirty garments thrown across the room in a messy pile, whose fumes drifted throughout the room. Each day she'd promised to clean up everything—furnishings, clothes, floors, kitchen—but she'd been too exhausted.

Keeping up the effort to maintain the basics of an organized life was starting to defeat her.

She kicked off her shoes, crossed to the bathroom, and turned on the shower before flipping the switch that unfolded the narrow bed from its niche in the wall. She sat down and struggled to remove her smelly clothing, then fell back across the mattress. Listening to the sound of pounding water, she imagined floating in a soothing warm-water pool. She drifted, drifted.

She awoke with a jolt. It was dark, and she was trembling. "Oh, no!"

A whiff of organ preservative reminded her of the aborted shower; she would have to reset the automatic shutoff and absorb the heavy penalty for exceeding her daily quota of water.

She rolled off the bed, turned on the lights, and snatched up the telelink. Someone finally picked up after the twelfth signal. She identified herself and held her breath.

"You're calling late again, Dr, Hidalga."

"I know, but—"

"Laya's finished her homework and she's already in bed. We've discussed this issue several times, Doctor. Nothing has changed. All of this is most disturbing to Laya's routine."

"Look, I know it's *your* school, but Laya is *my* daughter. I have to talk to her."

A few seconds elapsed before the school preceptor responded coldly, "No more than five minutes."

Zoe swallowed her anger; the fight wouldn't be worth losing the opportunity to hear her daughter's voice.

"Mom?"

"Sorry it's so late, sweetie. I fell asleep."

"Are you okay?"

"Just tired. We need a vacation, just the two of us."

"I wish I was there now, Mommy. I'd rub your back for you, like I used to."

"That would be so very nice."

"You promised we'd be together soon. I don't like it here."

"I know."

"Mommy, can't you just tell them we want to be together?"

"I will, I will. Soon! I miss you."

Zoe could barely hold her head up.

"Why can't you get another job so you wouldn't be so tired all the time?" Her eight-year- old daughter's voice turned petulant. "Why would anyone want to be a doctor, anyway?"

"Well, if I hadn't gone to medical school, I might never have met your father, and there would never have been a you."

"Oh, Mom! I would have been here whether you were a doctor or not."

Zoe laughed, then gasped as a bolt of pain stabbed through her middle. It crushed her breath. She collapsed onto the bed.

"What's wrong, Mommy?"

"It's…it's just late I need to take a shower, and—"

"You still miss Daddy, don't you?"

A flood of tears kept her from answering for a moment. Then it was too late.

"We'll have to hang up now, Dr. Hidalga," the preceptor interrupted.

"Just let me say goodnight, tell her I love her."

"Goodnight, Doctor."

* * *

Zoe twisted from side to side in a bed way too short for her five-foot-eleven frame. She could feel her bare feet dangling in the air while her tossed blankets lay piled in a heap on the floor. Each night she yearned for a decent-length mattress even though it could never fit into the wall space. Did it really matter? She was awake most of the night anyway, fighting bouts of sheet-soaking sweats and teeth-chattering chills.

This night was no exception.

In the darkness of the early morning hours, she rolled over, staggered into the bathroom, and sank onto the cold toilet seat. A wash of sweat covered her body; she was torn with spasms of explosive diarrhea. The pain expanded, grew worse until her back stiffened, her hands contracted into tight fists, and she spewed vomit across her arms and legs and onto the rough tile floor.

"God dammit!" she shrieked, gasping for breath. She hammered weakly on the walls of the small cubicle. "Stop it!"

Pounding fists echoed back at her.

It wasn't the first time Zoe had disturbed her neighbors' sleep in recent weeks. She took a deep breath to shut out any outside interference to her concentration; soon the spasms began to ease and she gained a weak sense of control.

She forced herself to clean everything. She fought back her revulsion at the sight and smells around her as she washed the bathroom. But no matter how hard she scrubbed, the stench of fear still hung in the air.

Zoe wadded her soaked sleeping garment into a ball and stuffed it into the waste disposer.

She was filled with self-hatred—hatred for the body that betrayed her, hatred that her immune system allowed a monster virus to invade and overtake her. Beyond that, she hated her lonely life, surrounded by neighbors who didn't even care enough to find out if she needed help.

She struggled to get back to her bed, where she collapsed and stared at the ceiling. Her anger slowly subsided, but the pulsating pain in her gut remained. Discomfort had become a constant companion for the past month, but she was lodged into denial, still refusing to fully accept the truth. She probably had the same disease that killed her husband two years ago.

Pain ate away at her resolve.

Forcing herself off the bed, she flipped on a small table lamp and stared at her image in the mirror across the room. Moving closer, she examined her face; healthy pink skin had been replaced with a ghostly pallor, and green-black smudges seemed permanently painted beneath her dark sunken eyes. And then there was her severe weight loss. Her skin hung in loose folds over her ribs.

Bones poked out so that she looked like a fossil, all soft tissue long gone. And her breasts, which had once been full and rounded, now rested like wrinkled bags on her chest. No one would ever believe the walking skeleton in the mirror was only thirty-eight years old.

She fingered her dull, stringy hair and remembered when it hung in soft waves that covered her shoulders like a gleaming black cape, a gift from her Spanish ancestors. A flash of memory brought images of erotic pleasure when her husband ran his fingers through the thick, long strands.

She also remembered the promise to her daughter to be together again.

She rested her head against the mirror and whispered to the disintegrating image, “You can’t die *now*. Can’t.”

Chapter 3

Organ Harvest Division
Complex Vessel Procurement Section

Seka Joraine's neck muscles tightened as she snapped on her protective gloves. The room's acrid chemicals, in large specimen containers scattered around the room, made her eyes burn and her skin itch.

I hate this. Hate my life!

She had to force herself to ease onto the high stool at her station and reach for the wrapped instrument kit that held most of her dissection tools.

A quick search around the windowless room revealed that every workstation was filled— none of the ten other doctors in her department were out sick.

They had recently lost one of the most competent vessel retrievers to pulmonary complications. Since it was a common affliction, no one talked much about it. What was there to say? The air was deteriorating, even under the protective domes, even with the air scrubbers. The constant sound of people coughing all around her told the story. Everyone's lungs were compromised.

Her fellow employee had been replaced within a day without any fuss or trouble.

How easily others dismissed him from all of their minds, from their consciousness. No one seemed troubled by the loss.

But it troubled Seka.

Wasn't that person worth even a sentence, some small expression of remorse? No one in the unit seemed to care that they'd lost someone close to them, someone they saw every single work day. Seka asked about him, but no one knew any of the details surrounding the cascade of events. She shouldn't have been surprised. Real friendships in the department were rare. These people were not her friends.

The instrument package rattled when she picked it up to

read the attached tag with the practical info—the department where the instruments belonged, date of sterilization and expiration, and the initials of the person who had wrapped the whole thing together. As if she gave a damn!

"You're late again, Seka," said the department manager, who seemed to appear out of nowhere. "Not an acceptable habit you've recently picked up."

"Sorry," Seka mumbled. She couldn't stop herself from staring at her superior's long, polished fingernails. They made her wonder which species of deadly bacteria or viruses resided under those obscene red shells. Even a casual outsider could see that, with those nails, she wouldn't able to dissect *anything* in the Organ Harvest Facility.

Seka flipped open the instrument pack and set it closer to her, pretending to ignore the woman so she could get to work.

"Emory Dutton wants to see you in Administration at ten."

Seka jerked around to stare into her manager's indifferent eyes. A sudden rush of blood pounded in her ears.

"I haven't done anything wrong. What does *he* want?"

"Better have that saphenous vein ready for grafting before you go. We've been running short of those things lately and some bigwig is due for coronary surgery first thing in the morning." The woman buffed her red claws on her sleeve and started to walk away.

"Personally, I wouldn't want to be in your shoes. I've heard tell Dutton's a nasty piece of work."

She tossed a final comment over her shoulder. "If I were you, I'd be right on the dot for that appointment."

Seka looked at the clock on the wall.

8:35

"I will be," she said, feeling weak.

She wanted to empty her mind, push away all thoughts of the coming meeting with Emory Dutton, but she couldn't. She'd also heard stories about the CEO. Who in Medicorp hadn't? He was supposed to be married but the grapevine told of how the head man would stroll through the departments in the different divisions of the Medi-Prog Corporation and openly choose the females he wanted. Women simply disappeared when they refused to go to bed with him. Gone! Not a sign of them.

Was that about to happen to her?

She gagged at the thought. Reaching into her table drawer, she pulled out an energy bar and broke it into pieces, then tossed them, section by section, into her mouth. She chewed carefully until barely a residue of flavor coated her teeth. Her stomach began to settle down with the food.

She pressed a button on the delivery cart an aide had parked next to her table. A large mid-leg segment was mechanically separated and pulled out and up from a grouping of ten, each wrapped and layered, one on top of the other. She clasped the leg firmly, lifted it, set it down, and immediately clamped it to the table by the knee and ankle. She knew the missing thigh and foot were probably in one of the other labs, in someone else's work cart.

Either that or someone is creating a Surgiclone for surgeons to practice on.

Surgiclone sounded as though it was an anatomical part cultivated from cells as a teaching aid so doctors could practice their skills. But Seka knew it was just another hacked-up segment from one of the specimen tanks.

The thought of the tanks gave her a sudden chill. The central rotunda of the building was filled with a thousand of them, at least it seemed that way. It was the first place she'd seen during her orientation in Organ Harvesting. She never forgot it.

Seka needed to get moving. She studied the partial limb she'd clamped to her table. Most times the disarticulations were accomplished by clean, sharp cuts. This segment had hanging ragged ends. Pieces of tendons and fascia dangled in strips from the bone, as though the saw had stalled midway, tearing up everything. She should have been used to seeing that kind of sloppiness; it happened often enough. But she didn't like it. She swallowed hard, took a knife from her kit, and cut away the extra tissue before checking the number stamped on the patella.

She compared it to the informational login on the

computer.

#785762

It matched.

She could tell from the condition of the skin, the tight musculature, the lack of bulging veins that this leg had belonged to a young person.

No venous insufficiency. No varicose veins.

She sliced open the derma along the calf muscle and cut into the bulging muscle. The tissue was a dead white; it was obvious everything but the venous vessel in this leg was meant to be destroyed, even the bone. This was a final stop for this body part—with Seka in the Vessel Retrieval Division of Medi-Prog.

After carefully digging around in the tissue, then opening and closing the dissection tool with rapid movements, she separated surrounding cellular material and released the saphenous vein from all the adjacent tissue that had hugged around it. The sought-after blood vessel was flexible and resilient, as expected. Seka carefully cut out a long tubular piece that would probably be used as a graft to bypass an artery that had formed an occlusion or was dangerously stenosed.

For years, she'd been able to empty her mind when she worked on various *donated* or cadaver body parts. She stripped the vessels for future grafting and tried to think of her work as something not only important, but necessary. She was helping someone to stay alive, to stay healthy.

Things had changed.

She started to have nightmares; she couldn't stop visualizing the people who might have lived with these blood-filled arteries and veins nourishing their own bodies. She imagined what they might have looked like if they were still alive. Were they beautiful or ordinary? What were their names? Who were they? What had happened to them?

She stared at the leg she'd just mutilated. Tears welled up and spilled down her cheeks.

The dead haunted her.

And she'd begun to have fantasies about killing herself,

ending her life the way her parents had. Quick. In the blink of an eye.

Both had been microbiologists. Everyone said Seka looked like her mother. Dark eyes, fair skin, pretty smile. Her father had been warm and kind, but when she thought of her parents, she always thought of her mother's laugh first. She. It was her mother who accidentally jabbed a deadly, contaminated needle deep into her own hand. She never said a word to Seka, never warned her that she was destined to die within two days. And her dad never said that he couldn't accept life without her. They gave their farewells to each other and he shot her, then himself.

Seka found them, their brains scattered across the pillows, along with a note pinned to the blanket. They apologized for her having to deal with the mess of their remains and explained why they were committing suicide. A shiver rode her spine as she relived that horrible moment.

Has it only been a year?

Seka glanced up at the clock again. It was 9:35. She'd finished the retrieval in one hour.

She stood and sealed the saphenous vein in a designated collection container and flipped a cleansing switch. The unit began to bathe the vein in a special wash that would be followed by the introduction of liquid nutrients and regenerative fluids. Then it would be ready for its final grafting destiny.

She looked at the clock one last time, rushed to start the scrub down of her worktable and station. An aide hurried to complete the job.

She'd been quick, but there was only enough time to wash up and catch a transpod for the ride to Medi-Prog headquarters, where she would face—and accept—whatever awaited her.

Chapter 4

Medi-Prog Offices
Emory Dutton's Office

Emory Dutton sat with his chin resting on steepled fingertips. He was in no rush to speak to the young woman sitting opposite him, at least until his stomach stopped rumbling from the excessive, if unappetizing, mid-morning snack he'd rushed through.

He could see why they'd chosen her for the job. The new chief of Desisto Processing would get a voluptuous package for an assistant. Even in an androgynous purple corpiform, she was eye candy. Dutton regretted not having seen her before she was tagged for this assignment.

He relished her obvious discomfort as he openly eyed her face, her body. He sniffed at the air, enjoyed the smell of her sexuality and her fear. Dutton remained silent as he stared at her generous breasts; he imagined how they would feel, how they would taste, how they would look if they weren't hidden. When he finally met her large pleading eyes, she quickly glanced away. Her hands nervously roamed across her lap, then down the sides of her thighs.

He stifled a belch and reached into his desk drawer for a couple of Syncarb tablets, chewed them slowly and methodically until there was nothing left but a slight bitter aftertaste.

"You must be pleased to be out of Organ Harvesting," he finally said, not really caring one way or the other.

"Yes, sir," she answered, her voice docile, compliant.

Her submissive attitude was definitely a point in her favor. Yes, she would do as she was told.

"I understand it's not a very pleasant place to work."

"No, it isn't."

"Uh huh," he grunted with a nod. "I suggest you remember that."

He watched her stiffen as her gaze flit from place to place around the room. Her body language oozed primal fear.

"Are there any questions about your assignment?"

"No, sir."

"Good. And is it perfectly clear, you are to report directly to me?"

"Yes, sir." She inhaled and exhaled quickly "What do I tell my supervisor in Organ Harvesting?"

He leaned across the desk and carefully mouthed each word, "You work for *me*, now. The people in Organ Harvesting are no longer your concern. Do you understand?"

"Yes, sir. I understand."

Dutton leaned back into his seat." The problem we face here, Dr. Joraine, is that Desisto, as I've explained to you, is one of our most sensitive ongoing projects. In fact, the future of the entire Corporit system is directly linked to it. At the risk of being repetitious, you will not discuss any of this, or anything else you learn, with anyone, at any time." He leaned forward again and stared her down, "Your life could depend on it."

Seka nodded. He could see she was beginning to have doubts about what she'd gotten herself into even though only a few minutes earlier she was very animate in telling him that it would make her happy to never dissect another human being again. She'd also confessed that she would incinerate every piece of Corporit clothing she'd ever worn in the harvesting unit if only to banish the smell of tissue preservative permanently.

Yes, she'll do what she's told.

"As background, I think you need to know that we've yet to retain a chief of Desisto Processing for more than six months."

"Is there some special reason for that?"

He hadn't expected that question and had no intention of answering truthfully. He was the only person who had complete knowledge of the defections and final sanctions connected with the position. The fact was, no one walked away from that slot alive.

"It's a highly stressful job. Your responsibility is to make certain our system is not put at risk if there is any new managerial weakness. You will report even the slightest deviation of Nathan Quinn's normal behavior. Professionally, socially, or sexually."

"I'll try," she said.

"You'll do better than that," Dutton said, jabbing at the air. "You will *do* it!"

* * *

Emory Dutton rode the express pod down to the first floor and stepped out the front door of the Medi-Prog Corporit building. His gaze lifted toward his penthouse office. He couldn't actually see the details of anything that high, at least not where the windows were, but he could visualize them, imagine the very spot where he stood day after day, looking across his city, San Francorp.

His elegant office was at the top of the huge building because of his accomplishments. *He'd* built a massive corporation with multiple medical divisions that ranked among the top money-makers in the global Corporit world. That gave him the ultimate satisfaction.

He looked around—the streets were mostly empty. It was a work day. Corporations frowned upon personnel away from their designated spots during work hours. That was no way to run a business.

And that's the way it should be.

Finally, he turned around and stepped toward the waiting limo. The driver stood by the open door until Dutton slid into the passenger seat.

"Thank you, Clinton," Dutton said when the driver was seated. After he was belted in, he automatically reached for a cut-crystal tumbler, held it up to the light to make sure it was spotless. The fact that it was seamlessly stored in a compartment that blended in with the dark, plush upholstery and vanished when the lid closed, tickled him. He could never fully explain it, but it was probably because it was like having a secret compartment. And it was no secret that he loved secrets. He laughed at his own humor.

Dutton filled the glass with two fingers of Alexandra Brandy and held the glass up to the light again, this time to study the caramel color before swirling the liquid and taking a sip. He savored the drink with his tongue and smiled at the way it made his teeth tingle. He inhaled the mellow fragrance, enjoyed the raw sense of power that swept over him.

"Are you comfortable, sir?"

"Quite, Clinton."

"Where would you like to go, sir?" "Take me to the James Complex."

The driver tipped his hat and pulled away from the curb.

Even Dutton recognized how childish and self-deceptive it was to take so much pride in something that could be wrenched away by taking one false step. But he couldn't help patting himself on the back; he hadn't made any false steps climbing to the top of his corporation. Many detours, but that was all they were: detours. But none that had derailed him.

When he started his rise within the Corporit structure many years ago, everyone trusted him. Not so much now.

Comes with the territory. Trite, but true.

He leaned back and stared out the window, continuing to savor the moment. He was one of the few CEOs permitted to have a luxury vehicle, along with Clinton at his beck and call. The aroma of the ersatz leather made him nod in satisfaction. Few things made him feel strong and potent the way having this car did.

He smiled. Actually, most things were his for the asking. And he only had to ask…once.

The only blight on the horizon was his sixtieth birthday. That mandatory retirement age remained an axe poised over his head. In two years, all of this would end. And what would he do then? Not much. There were no hobbies in his closet waiting to be pulled out and played with. Even with the remaining perks, he would mostly live in his own shadow. How could anything compare to the dominance that filled his life now?

Time had become his greatest enemy. Even he, with all his power, couldn't avoid the grim reaper, or the Corporit National Council retirement edicts.

He laid his head back and closed his eyes.

During the ride to his mistress's apartment he usually indulged in sexual fantasies about what was going to happen during the next couple of hours. Even though his wife Barbara knew all about his use of different women for his erotic pleasures; she remained silent.

Use of women?

Was that an unfair description? No. The term didn't bother him; that's just what it was. He used women to satisfy his every whim, every single desire. His wife had not only lost her beauty, but any sexual drive she ever possessed many years ago. All of that was a thing of the long gone past.

Why was he thinking of Barbara? This was the time he usually started imagining Taura slowly taking off her clothes, showing ripe breasts, puckered nipples, teasing, just out of reach of his mouth. He liked to think about that, not only what he would do to her, but even better, what she would do to him. A flash of her black eyes and moist mouth licking him always caused a feral stirring in his groin.

Out of nowhere, a sudden vision of Nathan Quinn's face jumped in and destroyed his special time. Not only Barbara, but the new Desisto Processing chief had edged Taura out of his reverie. Quinn had now lodged himself into the synapses of Dutton's brain like a rooted turnip.

He opened the liquor compartment again and refilled his glass. He didn't savor it this time. He downed the second brandy in one rapid swallow and, before he could stop, refilled his glass again, breaking a long-standing promise to himself never to have more than one drink before his session with Taura. Now he'd swallowed three performance-crushing drinks that even the latest pharmaceuticals couldn't offset.

Dammit! This is supposed to be my play time.

Discontentment cut through his bowels.

His inadequate, dull, lumpy wife, who spent more time

with their grown children than she did with him, continued to ride on Nathan Quinn's back. Together, they rummaged around in his head.

He visualized his wife: a tall, bulging, aging body spread out in all directions. Worst of all was her one unforgivable fault: her extreme disinterest in him. He couldn't remember when they last kissed. Barbara, his life's companion, avoided any physical intimacy with him, or anyone, as far as he could tell. She barely kissed their son and daughter when they visited, even though she looked forward to seeing them. He would have gotten rid of her years ago, but she knew everything about him, knew where all the bodies were buried—and he needed her cooperation, her silence if nothing else.

He started to feel a rush from the drinks, but as thoughts of his wife receded into the background, Nathan Quinn remained firmly lodged in his mind, combined with endless negative scenarios that made the hairs on his neck prickle.

Dutton had learned to trust his instincts, which took precedent, even over unrelenting logic.

Was it my imagination or is there something that's not quite right about that man?

Well, he was a Quinn, wasn't he? Or maybe it was because everyone he'd previously planted in that Desisto slot turned out to be a loser.

Every single one.

What was so difficult about the job? All anyone had to do was follow the statistics of population growth verses space available. It was a simple equation: when X and Y didn't match, Z became the only option. Cut the population. That's where Desisto took precedent. A simple equation. A child could not only do the math, a child could do the job.

What really vexed Dutton, what got under his skin about Quinn, was that he expected more humility, more deference from the people who headed up the many divisions in Medi-Prog.

He knew the man would continue to be a problem. But then, what else could he expect from a Quinn? It was in their genes. Dutton had almost turned Nathan down for the position on that alone. And he would have if he hadn't thought he could make good use of this Quinn by turning him into a pawn in his game of control.

Yet, barely into the job, Quinn started asking far too many questions about the ins outs and whys of Desisto.

Idiot! Just do the job!

He thought again about all the people who had been in charge of that division. None of them ever had the spine to do what it took to safeguard Corporit's existence. Like loose threads, they had been cut away.

Emory Dutton did not tolerate loose ends.

The car stopped and jolted him back into the present. He was now definitely in bad humor. The interlude he'd planned was spoiled. He was lightheaded from the alcohol and knew there would be no satisfactory, intimate sex.

He left the limo, took the elevator to Taura's apartment, refused to use the key. He pressed the buzzer to the suite without lifting his finger. The door sprang open. Taura took one look at him and quickly stepped back. The hand that flung out to slap her cheek missed its mark the first time.

But not the second.

Chapter 5

San Francorp
Noncorp Sector

Zoe hid in the shadows of a crumbling building at the edge of Corporit territory. She strained to make out the disintegrating letters on a rusted sign at her feet. If she was right, she was standing in the remains of a restaurant and bar she and Elliot had frequented years ago.

Flattening against the brick wall, she peeked around the corner at the main border crossing from San Francorp into the Noncorp sector.

San Francisco.

Zoe loved the sound of the original name, but the Corporit Wars had changed everything.

Countries around the world became subsidiaries of the International Corporit Council. Colorful cities, with their exciting historic images, were swallowed up, homogenized into ordinary names like San Francorp, Chicagocorp, Newyorcorp, Moscorp, Londoncorp.

She peeked at the border guards again. Even from her hiding place, the sounds of their heavy feet crunching loudly on a spread of glass unnerved her. No one could get near that fence without being seen or heard.

Zoe had gone over this moment time and time again. Now that she was actually here, could she work up the courage to approach the crossover, stand in the border's blinding lights, and withstand the scrutiny of soldiers with their guns drawn and ready to kill her?

The thought made her spine tingle.

She reached into her pocket, carefully pulled out two stimulant pills, and dry-swallowed them. That she'd begun to use more of the medication to get through each day worried her, but she couldn't take a chance on any unexpected weakness. The drug would help her function better—for at least a few hours—before she had to take more.

The sudden blast of a klaxon, with its shattering sound waves, made her jump. She covered her ears and stared at a huge holographic sign that appeared out of nowhere, was suspended in air, and flashed on and off in a brilliant red:

WARNING
ENTER THE NONCORP ZONE AT YOUR OWN RISK
RETURN NOT GUARANTEED
CORPORIT PAPERS MANDATORY

Her hands shook and breathing became difficult.

What am I doing here?!

What did she even know about Noncorp? The bits and pieces that she'd heard were frightening. It was a dangerous place. The one thing she did know; many of her friends who were forced into the zone were never heard from again.

She turned up the oxygen in her portable tank and took several deep breaths before she calmed down.

She would have to go now … or not at all.

Now!

She stepped out, heading straight for the guard at the gate. Her legs wobbled, her heart lurched in her chest, and she shook inside her insulated Zynec jumpsuit.

The glass under her feet alerted the nearest soldier. He spun around and pointed an electro-stun gun at her face until her sweaty fingers gave up her Corporit ID card. His wrist scanner covered the surface of the Ident-card as he waited for the information to verify that she was truly Dr. Zoe Hidalga.

She saw her goal in the distance: the reflected lights of the 24-hour Noncorp medical complex about a quarter-mile south of San Francorp.

"Are you sure this is what you want to do, Dr. Hidalga?" The guard pointed vaguely in the distance. "You may not be granted return privileges." When she didn't respond, he peered at her more closely. "Is something wrong?"

She shrugged, ignoring both his comment and the blinking red danger globes that marked the boundary between San Francorp and Noncorp.

"May I go now?"

The guard handed back her card, switched off the barrier shield, and waved her through, shaking his head. "It's your funeral, Doctor."

You've hit the nail on the head, soldier.

Today, she would finally face up to the truth, the presence gnawing away at her insides.

She stepped into Noncorp territory on the other side of the gate. When she looked around, she realized that Corporit may have squashed political ideologies, but had been no more successful in stopping the deterioration of the ecosphere than any other ruling system before them. The worlds on both sides of the barrier were falling apart.

She walked through the rubble toward the distant Noncorp Corporit Anatomical Resonance Examiner unit.

Ahead, shadowy, abandoned buildings stood between her and the Noncorp CARE towers. She knew that only ten years ago this area had been a thriving commercial spot of exclusive shops and expensive boutiques. Now it was eerie and vacant, filled with ominous silence.

Zoe stayed in the middle of the unlit street, keeping her distance from the derelict buildings on either side.

She sucked hard on her carry-all oxygen when her gnawing panic made her breath catch in her throat. Each footstep was loud, especially when she stepped on pulverized rock. And there was also the squish of things she refused to even think about. Stumbling over piles of debris, she kept losing her footing, and one time screamed at the shadowy outline of a dead body.

Male? Female? Did it matter? It was dead.

A sudden bolt of pain ripped through her gut. She doubled over. When it became bearable again, she continued shuffling forward, more determined than ever to reach the CARE facility.

She quickened her pace, hurrying toward the glow of light in the distance.

She'd taken no more than a few steps when her head was snapped back by rough fingers ensnarled in her hair. Her legs gave way and she was thrown to the ground.

"Hold her, dammit!"

A shapeless figure straddled her ankles. "She's too big, Godan!"

Twisting free, she lashed out and kicked the man hard in his crotch.

"Bitch!"

Her arms and legs were weak, but the stimulant had kicked in and she forced herself to sprint toward the bright lights ahead, shouting for help. The men caught her again and dragged over to a brick wall, pinned her against it. She was trapped.

"Get her fingers!" one of them shouted, jabbing a shoulder into her chest. The stench of him made her gag.

"Slice them off! Hurry!"

The other man struggled to pin an arm against the wall. With all her strength, Zoe smashed a heel down onto his foot. She spun around and sank her teeth into the grimy hand of the man with the knife.

"You idiots!" she screamed, spinning away from them. "You don't want my blood spilling over you. I have VMAS!"

"Son-of-a-bitch!" one of them shouted. He backed away, scampered over the wall.

Both men disappeared into the darkness.

Chapter 6

CARE Complex #2
Noncorp Sector

Stark black outlines silhouetted against the night sky. Thirty feet tall.

Windowless.

Ominous.

Zoe stared at the three lone structures. They stretched high above her on barren land, like giant aliens ready to pounce and absorb her flesh and blood. A bolt of fear rode her spine.

Run! Run! Run now!

No! I will not run.

Instead, she melted into the crowds that coiled around the CARE unit silos like a nest of crazy snakes she'd seen in the zoo when she was a little girl.

The National Council bragged about this Noncorp medical facility, and Zoe knew the Corporit Anatomical Resonance Examiners were medical powerhouses; self-contained robotic units that could examine and diagnose—even perform—surgery.

Her husband Elliot used to say, in the early days of Corporit takeover, "Providing access to CARE units to Noncorps is a cheap way to hold back rebellion. Shut them up. Shut up the poor masses and exiled Corporits by giving them something everyone wants: health care."

At least it *was* something.

And everyone in line wanted that something. They wanted answers. That's what Zoe was here for—answers to quell the doubts, confirm the unthinkable.

Corporits touted the CARE units as an example of health care generosity. Zoe had heard them brag often enough, heard the propaganda *ad nauseam*. She also knew that good will began and ended with the CARE units. All other transactions between the two entities were settled for cold, hard cash.

No exceptions.

The air was frigid; families huddled together to keep warm. Others stood alone, silent, pulling their coats and shawls tightly around them, shifting from foot to foot to keep their balance as the unrelenting wind pelted them. Over the hours, many fell asleep and slowly drifted away from their place in line. Not for long. They soon awoke and shuffled back to their spot.

She'd never met a Noncorp resident, and now she was surrounded by them. Some were easy to identify, such as artisans with smears and splatters on their clothing. Others were dressed in clean, but worn clothing. Everyone here was poor. Most were in bad health.

No one except Zoe wore insulated outerwear.

She heard the grumbles, meant for her ears, about the lying Corporit and its broken promises for a decent Noncorp medical system with real doctors and nurses—people they could talk to. But overriding their rebellious complaints were the harsher realities of coughing, wheezing, and the loud sucking of air on portable oxygen containers to avoid the ever-present pulmonary complications.

"You don't belong here," a Noncorp snapped behind Zoe.

"You can get *real* examinations, *real* treatments," another said.

Many turned to stare at her in her warm Corporit clothing. She spun around to respond, but the words died when she looked at an emaciated man's face—a mask of purple lesions that matched those under the sleeves of her suit. She scanned the crowd; about one in ten showed manifestations of the deadly VMAS virus.

And why *was* she here?

Because I'm a coward.

She couldn't bear to have a living, breathing Corporit medical counselor tell her face to face that she was infected with an untreatable disease. Zoe didn't want to look in their eyes and see her death sentence written there. She wanted an indifferent piece of machinery, a cold, heartless robotic examiner to confirm her own diagnosis.

A machine didn't care that she would die soon, never be with her daughter again.

She wrapped her arms around herself, tried to shut out the ugly leers and snide comments. She didn't want to think about it even though she knew the protesters were right. She *was* stealing a place in line, taking it away from a Noncorp, making every one of them wait longer.

All because I'm a coward that can't deal with reality.

Noncorp reality was different than hers. Reality here meant a harsh life filled with the constant struggle to survive. At least that's what she saw around her.

Wasn't it better to be a compliant Corporit instead of a political dissident that ended up in this place in the middle of nowhere?

Wasn't it better to have money? Stay with Corporit, work at two or three jobs, if one had to, so you could live within the safety of a controlled area?

The answers: Yes—to all her questions. And no matter what happened here tonight, she would never leave San Francorp again. She didn't belong with these people.

The sky was changing, getting lighter. It would be dawn soon. If she didn't enter the diagnostic unit within the hour, she would be late for work. This whole trip would have been for nothing.

Then, it was finally her turn to enter one of the CARE units.

Fear drained the blood from her head, leaving her dizzy and numb. She wanted to turn around and run back to her apartment. She stood paralyzed; unable to enter, unable to escape.

"Go!" urged a quavering voice.

A hand nudged her back.

Still she didn't move. The muttering became louder, more insistent.

What am I doing here? I deserve a health counselor. I'm a Corporit! "Suffering culture shock, sweetie?" a female voice chided.

Zoe was shoved through the open entry before she could change her mind. The door hissed closed behind her, sealing her within.

* * *

Her eyes squeezed shut.

When she dared open them, she realized she was in a compact chamber, much smaller than the exterior of the silo led her to believe. What had seemed ominous and frightening was in reality not much different from a small examination room.

She clamped her teeth to stop the erratic staccato clicks and clutched her arms to still her random quivering. Where was the equipment and complex robotics? There was nothing here.

Everything was hidden from view.

Luminescent pink light spilled around her. A warm yeasty smell filled the space and a sudden feeling of surrender, of total acceptance came over her. She took a deep breath, relaxed, and was infused with an unexpected sense of euphoria.

It was short-lived when she realized she was being manipulated into compliance.

The bastards are sedating me so a robot can tell me I'm going to die.

Shivering again, she waited in the dim light. She knew what the diagnosis would be. She had VMAS.

Viral Mal Absorption Syndrome. That was the virus that destroyed Elliot, almost without warning. And now she, too, was wasting away with the same disease that seldom allowed more than six months of life once the infection took hold. Half of her time was already gone.

She covered her mouth to keep from screaming.

"Please remove all your clothing," requested a computer-generated voice, shattering the silence.

Zoe stripped out of her Zynec suit. She'd never been shy about undressing before, but when she stood naked in front of a hidden computer, she not only felt vulnerable, it was as though she was surrendering her soul.

"Please place your hands over your head," the computer requested.

The lights went out and she was left in darkness until a panel of blue, purple, and green indicators blinked on.

She couldn't stop shaking.

"Place the second and third fingers of your right hand within the outlines of the DNA sensor on the panel in front of you."

Zoe did as she was told. She would soon have the answer.

"Thank you. Now place your fourth finger on the adjoining indent."

She winced as a minim of blood was quickly extracted from her fingertip.

"Please remove your hand."

There was the faint aroma of disinfectant; the floor began a slow rotation. She stiffened as soft tentacles brushed against her, touched every inch, every part of her body.

"Please describe your symptoms."

Her voice sounded weak and frightened. "Weight loss, abdominal pain, diarrhea, vomiting, skin lesions, hair loss, weakness, and constant muscular contractions."

The lights flashed, the machine whirred, the tentacles continued to assess. The entire examination took no more than five minutes.

The chamber light came on again. Zoe held her breath, staring intently at the dimming panel.

"You may dress, Dr. Hidalga. Rest assured, your symptoms will soon subside," said the pleasant, artificial voice. "We are pleased to inform you there is nothing wrong with you that requires treatment. Rx is deferred. Thank you for visiting CARE Unit Number two dash four zero seven."

As Zoe finished putting her clothes back on, the door behind her hissed open.

"What did you say?"

There was no response.

"You're wrong!" she yelled, backing out of the unit.

"You're wrong!"

Impatient hands shoved her aside.

The door to CARE Unit #2-407 slid shut.

Chapter 7

Cable Car Conglomerate
Corporit Singles Complex #25

The telelink's buzz startled Andrew Potter, shattering his concentration. He'd been pacing around his apartment after coming out of a long shower. He was still in the living room, memorizing his notes for a critical presentation later in the morning. A cup of real coffee, rare as champagne, sat on a small kitchen table, tempting him to stop and enjoy the moment.

But the telelink kept buzzing. The interruption not only annoyed him, it made him realize the importance of the meeting. The board would have to be convinced that financing his newest surgical robot was not only the best solution for the repair of traumatic neural damage available, but that the invention would mean hard cash in the bank for Medi-Prog. He had to convince those dull, corporate money-makers that this project was worth every cent of their investment. If he couldn't do that, there would be many, many more unnecessary deaths.

He thought of all the lost sleep, those late nights of hard work, pushing himself to the limits because he knew there was an answer.

And he'd found it. Dammit! He'd found it!

He grabbed the buzzing unit and pressed it to his ear.

"Andrew?"

"Who is this?"

"Andrew, it's me. Zoe Hidalga."

It took a beat to connect the voice with the name. He hesitated, eased himself into a chair. A sudden iciness raced through his body.

Few people had this number. There could be others listening. He had to be certain. One slip could destroy him. Destroy the others. He slowed his breathing and visualized Zoe and her daughter Laya, and his closest friend, Elliot. Yes. It was the voice of his lily-white friend, Zoe Hidalga. At least, that's how his coal-black mother used to describe her.

"Zoe! How are you?"

"I'm not sure. I just came back from a visit to a CARE unit."

Andrew's stomach clenched. "CARE? Why, for God's sake?" He was up and moving again, tight little steps from one end of his apartment to the other. He edged up to the room's window and watched the sun as it climbed higher in the sky. The city's amber dome shell darkened what used to be a golden globe of sunlight. Now, on most days, only a pinpoint of orange stared back at him through the layers of a carbon-filled atmosphere.

"You're a Corporit citizen, Zoe. You don't need to use one of those Noncorp machines."

She didn't answer immediately, then, "I have VMAS."

Andrew shook his head. "That's a CARE diagnosis?"

"No. But I know."

"Where are you now?"

"I just got back to my place."

"No!"

"Andrew?"

"Get out of there!"

Her voice was shaky. "I don't understand."

"You're in danger! Just do it! Get out! Now! Please!"

Andrew's mind was firing with questions but the answers would have to wait. He checked his watch. They couldn't have been talking more than a minute. Odds were in his favor that no one had tapped into his line at this hour, but the conversation could have been electronically recorded during a random check. The connection had to be severed.

"Meet me at the Corpmall coffee shop. East side. Half an hour." His voice was low and harsh.

"But—"

He hung up.

* * *

Andrew was shaken. His dead friend, Elliot, and his wife, Zoe, had been like family. Elliot had helped Andrew crystallize the goals of the Defy movement. In the beginning, both of them had put themselves at terrible risk to recruit the original resistance members. Believers whom they hoped would one day overthrow Corporit.

Someone had fingered Elliot and put him under constant surveillance right about the same time he came down with VMAS. On his death bed, he made Andrew promise that no matter what happened, he would never give up their battle to bring free choice back to the world. He'd also begged Andrew to look out for Zoe and Laya.

Andrew had kept his promise and the Defy followers were growing at an astounding rate. It was not only Corporit's abuse of power, which angered not only those who at one time were considered the middle class, but also many who were hidden within the upper power structure. It was apparent even to the dullest mind that the planet Earth was in its death throes.

Many Defys had been rabid nonbelievers of climate change when the movement started. But with the devastating increase of hurricanes, tornados, droughts, and other weather anomalies that were destroying the infrastructure of city after city, and the rapid destruction of plant and animal life, they were force fed the truth.

The final insult was their being shoved into enclosed cities. Denial was no longer an option.

Andrew had been extremely careful to stay within the parameters of Corporit life, while trying to protect the Defy movement.

But he'd let Elliot down. He'd been too busy to keep in touch with Zoe and Laya. Now, he would be forced to live up to his promise. He would have to try to save his friend, even though any action he took to help her could expose him.

* * *

Zoe plopped down on the edge of her bed. The stimulants she'd taken many hours earlier had metabolized out of her system. The trip to the Noncorp zone had not only left her wasted, it had left her confused. How could the CARE unit, a diagnostic wonder, declare there was nothing wrong with her? Impossible. She knew she was infected with VMAS.

The urgency in Andrew's voice buzzed in her head.

What's the matter with him?

Could she even get herself together to go out to meet him, or even go to work? She was exhausted and needed a hot shower and the emptiness of sleep.

But Andrew had been so insistent.

She slipped out of her filthy clothes. The fabric was heavy with the smell of her perspiration, mingled with the rancid odor of the men who'd attacked her. She tossed the soiled garments on top of the discarded clothes from the last few days and once again felt guilty for the mess.

She walked into the bathroom, eyed the shower, but settled for a splash of water on her face and underarms before pulling on fresh clothes.

"Damn you, Andrew Potter." He was Elliot's best friend; she'd called him for moral support.

Things were out of whack. First, the robotic machine lied about her physical status, and now her friend was acting…what? Nuts!

He'd not only hung up on her, brushed her off, but he was acting so crazy it scared her.

Still, the terror in his voice had been very real.

Why?

She parted the blinds and looked down on the street below. Two hovervans pulled up and settled down onto the pavement in front of her building. It was the police. The CAPOs.

"My God! He was right. How could he possibly know?" She stood frozen for moment, watching a squad of CAPO marshals jump out of the vehicles and fall into a tight military formation.

Then she turned away and ran for the door.

Chapter 8

Cable Car Conglomerate
Corporit Singles Complex #7

George Potek studied his action-ready marshals, all standing at attention. These were his people—the ones he personally chose to represent the Corporit Arms Protective Organization. They were the cream of the crop. They looked strong, capable, and more than ready to snap up any Desisto Processing candidate.

Should have stayed in the office. Especially since I have a shitload of paperwork to do.

But he couldn't help it. He wanted to be here, liked being in the field, in the thick of things. And he believed in a hands-on approach to leadership, even though he hated the pickups of DP losers. They were usually the whiners and screamers; they always made his nerves stand on end.

He remembered the first DP he picked up. The woman had gotten down on her knees, grabbed his leg, and begged him repeatedly to let her go. She pleaded for him to let her at least run to Noncorps. In the end, his marshals had to shoot her.

Messy.

Potek tried not to think about it. But Emory Dutton, with his gigantic Medi-Prog divisions, was his security company's biggest account. Desisto Processing was a big part of that corporation's operation. Losing Dutton's account would no doubt put him out of business. He couldn't afford to hate bringing in DPs.

Get it right or Dutton will nail my ass.

He eyed his marshals again. Everything from the tops of their heads to their Dunleavy boots was up to specifications. This was his elite group of officers and he was damn proud of them.

Annoyance disturbed his good humor when he noticed a problem with the bold lettering on one of the hovervans as it took off and peeled away—all of the *O*s in **CORPORIT ARMS PROTECTIVE ORGANIZATION** were defective and needed to be reapplied. Black had faded to gray.

Son of a bitch!

Well, someone would take a two-week pay cut for that lapse of detail.

It'll be fixed today or I'm not Commander George Potek.

He had to stay vigilant. It hadn't been easy for his CAPOs to become number one in the Tri Sector Area. And maintaining that status would be even harder. Other smaller security corporations kept trying to nip away at his leadership and his organization's motto: Security-Antiterrorism-Profit.

So far, the CAPOs were by far in the lead. No one was even a close second when it came to security. In fact, if anything, the competition had been falling by the wayside like dead flies.

That only reminded him of how complicated his life was becoming. This morning he had been called before his CEO and the Board of Directors to further explain new costly operative maneuvers. Potek had been realistic and thorough. He couldn't be absolutely sure, but he thought he still had their confidence. But the bottom line always seemed to win out over practicality and reason.

He'd better not let them down. He liked his job.

Potek sensed the CAPO marshals were growing restless. They had their tasers holstered, but their fully automatic Sydarms 10mms were at the ready, and the group had formed a tight circular defensive position.

Alert.

Silent.

Menacing.

The moment they'd arrived at the apartment complex, the handful of people walking down the street vanished almost in a blink of an eye. It always amazed him that the CAPOs had that instant effect on the good citizens of San Francorp. The observation never failed to bring a rush of pleasure as he watched everyone move out of their way, fear etched on their faces. That kind of power was addictive; he never got enough of it.

All eyes were riveted on Potek. He finally signaled the marshals to enter the apartment complex.

"Keep those god dammed tasers in your holsters and your guns on safety unless I tell you otherwise," he ordered in a gruff voice. He did a close-up inspection of each of their red Zynec jumpsuits and shiny Polytek helmets as they marched single-file past him. *A-one, dammit!*

When they entered the building, two tenants about to leave turned quickly and ran back down the long hallway, hissing a nervous warning, "CAPOs. CAPOs!"

Potek and his marshals squeezed into a large, square vaculift and shot upward nonstop to the nineteenth level. Their footsteps clacked a hollow echo on the ebonite floor. They walked quickly toward Zoe Hidalga's apartment. Potek fully expected to catch her before she left for work.

Standard operating procedure was to avoid nabbing a suspect at his or her job—poor PR. Other workers would become uneasy, make them think of the "D" word—Dictatorship. When it did become necessary to go to the place of employment, it was considered poor planning. It usually meant a black mark against the leader of the unit.

"Dr. Hidalga!" the commander shouted, pounding on the thin door. "Commander Potek from Corporit Arms! Open up! Open up now!"

When there was no immediate response, he banged on the door again and looked up and down the empty corridor. He turned to a female marshal standing next to him.

"We never seem to draw a crowd, do we?" It was closest he ever came to humor. He checked his watch, waited exactly sixty seconds.

"Open the door, Dr. Hidalga!"

Without waiting for a response, he unlocked the door with

a passkey, indicating that the marshals fire on contact, if necessary.

Each marshal released the safety on his weapon.

Can't say I didn't provide the opportunity for her to do this peacefully.

Potek gave a *do it* motion with one hand, then stepped aside to allow his marshals to rush into the apartment.

"She's gone!" one shouted.

"Damn it!" Potek said, entering the small, cramped living quarters. He was disgusted at having to spend more time finding the diseased woman. This kind of thing always made him look incompetent, especially when the pickup should have been a piece of cake. He quickly looked around, nodded, and said, "Strip it! You know the procedure."

He stomped out, leaving the follow-up details to his marshals. In less than an hour, they would empty the apartment, leaving behind no sign of Zoe Hidalga.

As Potek left, he heard the excited neighbors on either side of the doctor's unit talking to one another through cracked-open doors. They thought the six-day fumigation process of Hidalga's unit might be even worse than her frequent nighttime disturbances. But they really seemed more curious about who would be the new occupant.

* * *

Across the street from the apartment complex, hidden in a doorway, Zoe watched and trembled as all of her furniture and personal belongings were loaded into a hovervan.

Hot tears streamed down her cheeks. The marshals carried out the few paintings she and Elliot had spent long hours selecting, and she knew that buried in the cartons were the only existing pictures of her husband and daughter.

They'd not only taken her few possessions, they'd stolen her family.

Laya!

What was going to happen to her?

Zoe wanted to dash out, confront them, kick and scratch,

wrestle the boxed remnants of her life from their hands. But she remained hidden, fists clenched at her sides while the stuffed vehicle drove away and disappeared from view.

Chapter 9

San Francorp
DP Processing Division Medi-Prog Offices

Nathan Quinn was stunned.

There's a name I haven't seen in years.

He leaned back into his chair and studied the computer screen. In a long column of overnight DPs, his eyes fixed on a single name: Zoe Hidalga.

"I don't believe it!"

His new executive assistant, Seka Joraine, walked through the open doorway.

"What's wrong?"

Nathan turned away from the overnight report for CARE Unit #2-407, ignoring Seka by looking out the window at the adjacent office building. It was close enough that he could watch the office workers move around in their cubicles. Sometimes when he watched them interact, walk from place to place, he wondered what they were saying to each other. But not today. Today he had no time for distractions. What he saw made him sad.

"A friend of mine has been black-flagged," he finally said.

"Who is it?" she asked, stepping toward his desk.

He waved her away. "It could be a coincidence or an error."

"Would you like me to check it out for you?"

"No, no," he said. "I'll look into it myself."

"You can't take every black flag personally."

Nathan was annoyed with her. "I know, but this isn't just *any* black flag. If it's who I think it is, we were schoolmates, close friends, and we lived only a few doors from each other."

"I see."

But she didn't see. He could tell she really didn't get it at all. Her unemotional response irked him in the same way he found himself irritated by the "so what" attitude among his fellow Corporits. It was like they were all involved in a complicated game and the contest was more important than the players.

He bit down on his lip. He'd already said too much. He'd had this position for only the last month and the idea of forced euthanasia was a lot more tolerable as an intellectual exercise rather than dealing with the actual statistics all day long. And Zoe was DP listed. It was becoming personal.

Seka had just become his assistant. He hardly knew her and couldn't risk her reporting him; the last thing he needed was to end up on some kind of blacklist.

"Would you please bring me the follow-up report on yesterday's Desisto Processing designees?" he asked.

"The new DPs, or the terminated ones?"

"Both," he said, noticing how well she had adapted to her new position.

When she was gone, he immediately turned back to his workstation and called up Zoe Hidalga's Persfile on his monitor.

Zoe Hidalga

Born: February 18, 2012

Education: Embarcadero H.S. Honors 2030 Embarcadero University, B.S. Biology 2034 Approved for Medical School Quota 2034 Corporit Medical School #15, Grad 2038 Internship: Corporit Harvesting, 2038-2039

Assignment: Staff, Organ Harvesting Unit, 2039 to date

Family History

Mother: Ardis (nee Lutz), Professor, Embarcadero University, Corporit Political Science
Deceased, heart disease
Finalized (DP 2048)

Father: Luis, Soils Engineer, Agricorp
Deceased, minor cerebral hemorrhage
Finalized (DP 2042)

Siblings: None
Blood Relatives: Few, scattered
Marital Status: Married 2039, Widowed 2048
Spouse: Elliot Woler, Physician-Gerontology, Medicorp Deceased, VMAS
Finalized (**DP** 2048)
Children: One (1), Laya, female, B2042

Social Profile
Well adjusted; reliable team member until spousal termination.
Carewatch alert 2048 (See spousal **DP** entry)
See disposition of offspring, Laya
Medical History
Appropriate vaccines Appropriate menarche Acceptable illnesses

Nathan was amazed at the amount of information available to him since his recent promotion. He took one of his frequent looks at the new identification plaque poised on the end of his desk:

NATHAN QUINN - CHIEF
Medical Programmer/Desisto Processing

When he turned back to the frozen computer image of Zoe's file, he found it troubling to see that both Zoe's mother and father had been Desisto Processed.

Wonder if Zoe knows anything about their final termination. Doubt it.

Why *had* he and Zoe drifted apart? They'd had real history together, were close friends until she married. Then they'd lost touch with each other.

She'd been very special to him. Even now, the more he tried not to think about Zoe Hidalga and that one idyllic summer, the more embedded it became in his mind. He couldn't forget her. She was always there, lodged in his memory, like a computer file stowed away and ready for future review.

Waiting.

* * *

Zoe and Nathan had been sixteen, a time when youth and longings seemed more important than any Corporit rules that controlled their environment, such as, *Amendment IV, Corporit Charter, 2028 – minor neighbors and schoolmates are not to vacation together. Corporitology studies reveal excessive fraternization among minors leads to cliques and misalliances detrimental to future efficient adult occupational functioning. Behavioral disturbances and adjustment failures are rampant, with unpredictable outcomes.*

A simple computer glitch bypassed the new Corporit edict and they *were* assigned to the same summer camp facility for twenty-five hundred youths in the Sierra. It might have been days or weeks before they found each other among the twenty-five hundred attendees that year. But they spotted one another the first evening at dinner. They expressed secretive smiles of recognition across the massive dining hall.

At a get-acquainted dance the same evening, the two acted like strangers. No one would have suspected they were from the same neighborhood, or had shared classes together the past couple of years. They circulated, chatted, danced with other partners, putting off the moment when they would *accidentally* meet.

The mixer had less than half an hour to go when Nathan moved into position to "introduce" himself to Zoe. When he asked her to dance, her dark eyes lit up, and his heart pounded into a gallop.

Zoe Hidalga had been his first love. They danced and playfulness blossomed into something unexpected. Her touch made his skin come alive and he surrendered to the thrill of holding her close to him. Even after all this time, he remembered how her perfume made him feel.

It almost kept him from breathing.

As they danced and talked, he wanted to be clever for her; but he couldn't speak. All he was able to do was move to the rhythm of the music and his inner longings.

* * *

Seka Joraine interrupted, brought Nathan back to the moment. He thought his heart would stop as he quickly body-blocked the screen so she couldn't see Zoe's Persfile.

Nathan knew it would be a serious mistake to spend any more time with Zoe's file, at least for now. He would have to return to it later, find some way to help her, do something about the black-flag death sentence.

He glanced back and forth between the screen and Seka, but as he started to clear Zoe's file, the computer announced that Zoe was now beyond anyone's help.

VMAS confirmed; CARE Unit #2-407
NONCORP ZONE
16 Jan 2050
DP ACTION COMMENCED

Nathan's chest constricted, tears clouded his eyes. The edict flashed across the screen:

DESISTO DESISTO DESISTO

Chapter 10

Cable Car Conglomerate
Corpmall #1

The cafeteria was jam-packed. A few hundred people were hanging out, putting off the moment when they would have to leave for work. An animated crowd created a constant buzz of conversation as people grabbed last-minute drinks, snacks, sandwiches, doughnuts.

Almost without exception, each person wore department color-coded corpiforms. Electronic IDs hung around their necks so that they could be scanned for immediate identification. A blur of green, blue, and yellow swirled around the food dispenser islands as everyone hurried from place to place.

After standing around for ten minutes with two steaming cups of corpcaf, Andrew Potter snagged a seat at one of the smaller tables. He sank into a molded Polytek chair and shifted his lanky body several times before he found a comfortable position. As he waited, he took small sips from his cup.

He was restless as he stared at gun-exchange posters plastered along the walls, almost like wallpaper that read: *Be legal. Exchange guns for food.*

Most guns had been turned in or collected long ago. But one of the few ways left to get rid of any hoarded weapons, other than by direct home inspection, was to offer an exchange for food.

It was easy to spot the undercover security guards intermingled in the crowds. Even though they sat at the tables, dressed in different department corpiform colors to blend in with the other workers, they were anything but anonymous. It was their peculiar habit of evaluating each person for only a minisec that gave them away; their eyes resembled bouncing balls as their gazes jumped around the room. It looked pretty funny to

Andrew. He wondered who had thought up that particular maneuver for a visual scan. It was idiotic and very noticeable.

And was anyone fooled by their *cleverness*? He doubted it. Probably everyone in the room knew they were CAPO spies, and why they were there. Nevertheless, their presence was a blatant warning: act up and you'll find yourself dealing with the security system.

And it worked.

Multiple acts of defiance every week had dwindled down to a trickle since the undercover guards were planted in the crowds. The café used to be a *really* noisy place, especially when so many people clustered under one roof. Now, the sonic level was just a buzz and the only raucous byplay this morning came from some teenagers in the back of the room.

Andrew sipped his bitter pseudo coffee, reading the electric neon news strips circling the room. The latest Corporit propaganda for the masses:

AUGHT OUTLAWS BREAK THROUGH CORPORIT PERIMETERS—ATTACK CORPORIT WOMEN AND CHILDREN—CAPO SECURITY UNITS KILL INTRUDERS—NONCORP LEADERS TURN DOWN CORPORIT FINANCIAL AID—ALARMING SPREAD OF VMAS IN OLDER POPULATION—

Where are you, Zoe?

If she didn't come soon he would have to leave. He was scheduled to demonstrate his newest neural repair technique at ten. He had to be there.

But there was so much he wanted to tell her, so much she needed to know.

He took another sip of his now-cooled corpcaf and brushed imaginary lint from his gray slacks. At least he didn't have to wear the designated maroon colors of the Robotic Division. Executives were freed from uniform requirements and other dress restrictions; one of the perks of being at the top of the heap.

Why had Zoe even gone to a Noncorp CARE unit? Still, it was lucky she hadn't visited one of the Corporit medical counselors or it would have all been over.

Why hadn't she come to him first?

Working in Organ Harvesting has kept her too isolated, too naïve. He assumed she never dreamed Corporit would closely monitor Noncorp units.

But still, what was in her head? He couldn't imagine what she was thinking…or if she was thinking at all.

What if she didn't get out of her apartment in time? What if the CAPOs have already grabbed her?

Well, that would be it. There'd be no helping her. Any attempt on his part to reverse the DP process would bring the whole system crashing down on him and his covert operation. He couldn't endanger the lives of the Defys just to save one person.

He was convinced that Asher Wind Storm's network of survivors and the Defys *had* to succeed.

Someone slipped into the chair beside him. He turned and for a moment wasn't sure the woman staring back at him was Zoe. Her dark hair hung in limp clumps and her sunken eyes flashed anger.

"How did you know they were coming?" Zoe asked, almost demanded.

Andrew covered his shock at seeing her skeletal appearance by taking her hands in his. The contrast between her almost transparent paleness and the walnut shade of his black skin was stark.

"Zoe, I had to get you out of your apartment, but had to assume they might be recording all your conversations. There wasn't time for explanations."

"Then tell me now, dammit! How did you know?"

"Because you have VMAS," he said, indicating the purple splotches peeking out from the sleeves of her shirt.

"No one knows that but me…and now, obviously you."

"Zoe," he said softly. "you went to a CARE unit."

She snatched her hands away from him. "And it told me I

was healthy!"

He scanned the room, looked at the closest security guard, who was staring surreptitiously at them.

"Please calm down, drink your coffee."

Zoe looked at him, her eyes wide. "Andrew, I don't even know what kind of a mess I'm in. Or why. And those CARE units, are they dysfunctional? What's been going on while I've been stuck in that stinking organ-harvesting hole?"

"There are many advantages to not knowing the truth," he said.

"People who lie to you always say that. Name me one advantage." She straightened in her chair and yanked her sleeves down to cover the exposed lesions. "How does anyone know I have VMAS? I never saw a medical counselor. And, again, your robotic CARE unit said I was healthy."

"The unit lied. The minute you stepped into that CARE unit you were black-flagged for immediate extinction." Andrew looked away.

"Look at me, Andrew! Black-flagged? They're going to kill me?" Her eyes seemed to sink farther into their sockets. "And how do *you* know that, Andrew?"

"I'm the chief robo-surgeon, remember? I program the damn things."

Zoe shoved backward, crashing into the table behind her. "You miserable—"

"Lower your voice, Zoe," he whispered. "Now! You're attracting too much attention. Shrug it off and smile. I mean it! Do it now or I'll have to turn you in myself."

Zoe forced a smile. She reached for her corpcaf and pretended to sip the disgusting brew.

He could see she let the cooled drink remain in the cup.

"How did this happen?" she asked.

"The global Corporit National Council made the final decision. VMAS and all other terminal conditions have become too expensive for techno-maintenance. CNC hired Medi-Progs and their Desisto Processing Division to handle the solution … at a cost of billions of dollars, I might add. It's immediate termination upon detection."

Zoe slapped him across the face. "What kind of person have you become to get involved with something like this? You're supposed to be a doctor, not an executioner."

Andrew rubbed his face, let his shoulders sag. He glanced at the breakfast crowd. All eyes at the surrounding tables were on the two of them. He gave the diners and security a try-to-understand smile.

Grasping Zoe tightly by one arm, he hurried them out of the busy cafeteria. He didn't stop until they reached the water fountain in the center of the mall. There was no sign of water coming from the spigots on either side.

"Zoe, I don't have time for explanations right now. There's a lot more going on here, more than you can imagine."

She wrenched her arm away. "We've been friends for more than fifteen years, Andrew, but right now I don't know you…maybe I never did."

"You have to trust me, Zoe."

"Why should I?"

"Because I'm the only hope you have of getting out of the city alive."

Zoe sat on the fountain ledge. "I don't want to get out of the city. Why can't they leave me alone? I'm going to die anyway."

He sat down beside her, put an arm around her shoulders and hugged her to him. "Listen," he whispered. "It's not as grim as it appears. There are things going on…good things. Before he died, Elliot was part of it."

"Part of what?"

"The Defy network."

"The outlaw group? That bunch that's trying to overthrow Corporit? He couldn't have been; I would have known. Elliot was a healer, not a revolutionary."

"He was as involved as I am. Both of us worked from inside the system to undermine Corporit power, bring them down, get back to some kind of democratic elective process. And if we don't regenerate our environment—"

"How many others are involved?"

"I'm not willing, or allowed, to share that information. All you need to know is that each one of us has a specific role. It's safer that way."

She looked at him with tears spilling down her cheeks. "What am I going to do, Andrew? What's going to happen to my daughter after I die? She'll be all alone…she'll think her mother deserted her." Zoe sagged, leaned hard against him.

"Listen to me, Zoe—"

"And I'm so tired, Andrew. So very tired. I'm just not up to playing hide-and-seek with the CAPOs."

"Zoe, please! Listen to me! I can stop the VMAS and I can hold off the CAPOs. That's why I have to get you away from here."

"What do you mean you can *stop* VMAS?"

He sighed, looked around before he spoke. "There's a stabilizer."

"*Who* has a stabilizer?" she whispered.

"The executive staff has had exclusive access to one for almost two years."

"And you can get it for me?"

"Yes!"

She struggled to her feet. "You black son-of-a-bitch! You could have saved Elliot and you let him die!"

Chapter 11

Medical Programming Corporation
CEO Office Suite

"What do you mean the CNC turned me down?" Emory Dutton said.

"They reviewed your security goals," CAPO Commander Potek said, "and you need to fall in line with all the other corporations in the Tri Sector Area."

"Corporit National Council…Corporit International Council, my ass. Who the hell are they to tell me how to run my business? What a bunch of losers." Dutton pointed a finger at Potek. "*I* run this corporation and all of its medical divisions, and if I need their input, I'll ask for it."

"But, sir, Corporits have all agreed that the CNC would be the supreme overseer of every business. The council has the final word, and every corporation is bound by that agreement, including Medi-Progs."

Dutton glared at Potek. "You know I wasn't one of those who voted for that kind of all- inclusive authority. I don't like anyone looking over my shoulder." Dutton yanked a handkerchief out of his pocket and blew his nose. "I thought we got rid of governments and their nosy and interfering regulations thirty years ago."

"Sir, I respectfully submit that some oversight is necessary." The commander resumed reading his presentation to Dutton.

Dutton looked at George Potek's smooth, unlined face and trim athletic body. It immediately triggered thoughts about the sixty-year-old mandatory retirement age again. When he'd been Potek's age, he had no interest in the CNC age edict other than thinking it was an excellent idea. Now, at the other end of the equation, his appreciation had bottomed out.

He shifted a pile of papers from one corner of his desk to

another, studied the new arrangement for a moment, then repeated the process all over again. When he was finally satisfied, he stood and walked to a large corner window, his steps muffled by steel-gray carpeting that stretched from wall to wall.

He wasn't a patient man, but he tried very hard to concentrate on the security briefing the CAPO Commander—who sat rigidly in the chair across from his desk—was delivering to him. It was getting more and more difficult by the second.

At his best, Potek was irritating. Every point, major or minor, received equal emphasis. Without paying close attention, it was difficult to choose what *was* really important. Worse, he disliked the pragmatic CAPO commander, as much for his youth as anything else.

Potek was pointing at an info board. Everything was written in bold black letters. An updated CNC management and security system's schematic stared him in the face. Potek read from it aloud.

"*Corporit Community Control Update*

"One—Population Management: All aspects proceeding as planned. Desisto Processing (DP) will remain the primary measure of population control.

"Two—Fear Factor: Terrorist propaganda—satellite and private communication monitoring increase per CNC instructions.

"Three—Defy Identification: Numbers unclear, but group's active rebellion within the Corporit establishment is increasing with covert acts of sabotage. This will not be tolerated. All so-called Defys are to be treated as terrorists; punitive measures will be extreme. A special task force has launched investigations.

"*Noncorps Update*

"One—Central Noncorp committee still refuses to consider Corporit goals. This is not acceptable. In-progress plans will alleviate this problem. CARE units will be removed if compliance is not accomplished.

"Two—Reviver Population: Expanding under Asher Wind Storm, but at this time will be dealt with solely by the CNC.

"*Aughts Update*

"One—Leaders: Godan and Tabo only members identifiable to date.

"Two—Homeless population: out of Corporit and CNC control.

"Three—Terror attacks: These will not be tolerated. Immediate trial. Immediate capital punishment mandatory with guilty verdict. No appeal—"

Dutton interrupted with the wave of one hand. "Remind me about the Revivers again, Potek."

The commander, halted in mid-sentence, saw that Dutton obviously was annoyed. He flipped open his portable network and tapped a few keys to display his private notes on the big screen.

"As I've said at the past two briefings…" Potek paused to let that sink in. "... Asher Wind Storm is an indigenous person. This Indian is the most identifiable leader of the Revivers. They are a global group that moves into desolate areas worldwide and claims to regenerate extinct flora and fauna with Storm's Caplac domes. Oxygen for the Noncorp population is supplied by the Revivers. And we purchase most of our food for the Corporit population from the Asher Wind Storm agricultural network."

"And they claim those domes of theirs are not only growing food but generating enough oxygen to dispense to their population?" Just thinking about not having oxygen made Dutton breathless for a moment.

"This Indian and his group live among the Noncorps and he appears to have unexplainable success…almost magical, some claim." He stopped to bark out a short grunt. "He is regenerating species of plants and animals in his gigantic domes—the very same species that have been dying out since the twentieth century. This Maricopa mystic is also supposed to have unexplained healing powers—"

"Well, isn't he the wonder. Is there anything he can't do?" Without waiting for a reply, Dutton added, "Can we duplicate his successes?"

"There's been no success thus far after several attempts. Even when we use identical revival techniques, the results are negative. As things stand, we need him and his network."

"If he's that good, why hasn't he healed VMAS?" Dutton said dryly.

Potek shrugged.

"Have you personally interviewed this Maricopa? This Storm?"

"I've questioned him several times when he's entered the Corporit zone on business."

"Business?"

For the first time, Potek broke into a smile. "Ironic, isn't it. He also designed all the domes protecting San Francorp."

Dutton turned away from Potek and stared out the window. Being on the top floor of the Medi-Prog Corporation building, he looked at the only thing between him and the sky—the protective dome.

This Indian could shut us down. He has much too much power.

"How old is this Indian?"

"His age is undetermined, sir."

"We've been putting up these dome protectors for more than twenty years."

"His father created the original process," Potek said. "Storm continues his work and has improved on the basic concept. As you can see, we really need the man. We pay him large sums of money for the domes that protect the city, and with all the food he produces…he's almost untouchable."

"No one is untouchable. Put him on the CAPO watch list?"

"He's already on the list, sir. And we keep trying to track him." Potek chose his next words carefully. "But…he seems to vanish right before our eyes."

"Do better!"

"We'll try, sir."

"Yes, you will, Commander…or else!"

* * *

Dutton looked out the window, studied the way the surrounding see-through amber plastin dome underplayed the complexities of the intricate engineering.

He knew his Medi-Prog Corporation, and all of its divisions, had been the first to receive and install its own domes, to protect the vital profit center with all its highly trained professional people and critical services from the deteriorating global environment. Since then, every other Corporit profit center had received the domes, or were wait-listed.

He had been a young executive when they first started building the domes. Yes, it was easy to remember the date; right after the Corporate Wars of 2020.

Potek's voice became a background buzz to his thoughts.

Everything was in flux; decreasing productivity, worldwide drought, famine, diminishing forests; a dying environment. All of it seemed to escalate at once, and it worked in their favor. It was amazing how easy it had been for the Corporits to globally unite and squash governments at every level. That's when the Corporit International Council became the world's governing organization.

Almost overnight, central, state, and local governments were taken over and dissolved; corporate MBAs were assigned to stem the chaos, put things in order. They set up and organized the Corporit National Council to govern, and to operate individual corporate domains.

It wasn't really that difficult to edge governments out nationally and globally after they became so corrupt, bankrupt, impotent, and unpopular.

"As to the Aughts," Potek said "They—"

"Just a bunch of terrorist vermin to be exterminated," Dutton said. "Not much else to do."

"Excuse me, sir, but their raids in both our sector and the Noncorp sector continue to give the impression the CAPOs can't handle the job of protecting Corporit productive citizens."

"Tell me, Commander. What would we do without the Aughts? Fear of the terrorists is one of the things that make the population controllable," Dutton said. "It's what feeds Infocorp and its propaganda machine. Remember that, Potek."

"But it isn't easy to deal with, sir."

"It's *your* job. It isn't supposed to be easy." Dutton was really annoyed. Even Potek wanted everything easy.

What's the younger generation coming to?

"Whatever you need to do, *do* it!" Dutton shouted. "Besides, sooner or later, VMAS will finish that mangy lot. Then we'll be rid of them." He gave Potek and a dismissive flick of the hand.

"I'm more worried about the Defys," Potek said, "These people are Corporits, and they want a more inclusive society."

Dutton kept hearing more and more about the rebel group. Their activities kept floating to the top of Corporit's agenda. The CEOs were starting to really worry about them.

"What the hell do they really want?" he asked.

Potek looked thoughtfully at Dutton. "They want everyone to have more of a voice in the way our society is managed."

"I get that part. But I think what they really don't like is the harsh CNC rules." Dutton barked a laughed. "Well, you tell these misfits, neither do I. But you and I know someone has to have the last word or society will disintegrate into chaos."

"From what I've heard, they want Corporit to consider every segment and class of our society, not just the wealthy."

Dutton pointed at Potek. "And how do you know so much about what these outlaws want? Maybe you're one of them? It certainly sounds like you agree with them."

"It's my job to know," Potek said with just the edge of a smile at the corners of his mouth. "I don't agree or disagree. I just do my job."

Dutton turned away from the commander.

I need to look further into these rebels, not rely on underlings like Potek.

"Well, good luck to them. If they can get enough Corporits to get off their asses to start a revolt, then we deserve what we get."

"I think you underestimate them," Potek said.

"I don't underestimate anyone, Commander." Dutton stared at Potek until the man shifted in his seat.

They had been at it for more than an hour now, covering everything from building lockup security to CARE sabotage. Dutton was becoming more and more distracted; it was past time for his personal assistant to bring his midmorning tray. Dutton made it his business to eat something every two hours or his glucose bottomed out. He looked at his watch and visualized real coffee with the frosted Danish he'd requested. His stomach was starting to rumble, a sure sign that if he didn't eat soon, waves of nausea would commence.

Dutton shifted his short squat body in his desk chair, ran fingers through his freshly clipped gray hair. He wondered when Potek would finally finish his report. He began to toy with his pencils. He paused and stared at Potek, once again taking the measure of the man as he commenced reading again from his report.

He nodded absently at Potek and sat up straighter at his large, teak desk, one of the last in all the Corporit offices. Dutton didn't particularly like Potek, but he was good at his job…and he followed orders to a tee. The CEO sighed audibly, feigning interest in the continuing flow of words that were beginning to put him in a dream state.

"—routine investigation of Nathan Quinn, the new chief of Desisto..."

Dutton snapped to attention "Repeat that!"

"What?"

"The part about Quinn."

"Uh…Nathan Quinn, a Medi-Prog, recently named to head the depopulation project, also known as Desisto—"

"Get on with it, Potek. I know all the labels and titles. I helped create them. Just tell me more about Quinn."

The barest hint of a frown creased Potek's youthful face. He started again. "The CAPOs are conducting a routine investigation of Nathan Quinn, the new chief of Desisto

Processing."

"How long has he been on the job now, a month? Longer?"

"Thirty-five days."

"Anything suspicious?"

"I have been particularly cautious with Nathan Quinn, as you suggested, sir. He has not been an outstanding figure in the medical community. He's mostly worked with auxiliary medical units."

Dutton interrupted. "Which corporation?"

"Our corporation. Medi-Prog."

"I know the name of our corporation, Potek."

Potek continued as though he hadn't heard Dutton. "But he has limited himself to dealing with mostly statistical evaluations. That, and he's also been in charge of a number of medical supply outlets." Potek stopped for a moment. "Maybe his parents' reputation has overshadowed his progress."

"That man could have been anything he wanted," Dutton said. "I wonder why he chose that offbeat path?"

"Supplies and statistics seem to have been more in line with his interests since the completion of his internship."

"Not exactly a medical asset to the Quinn family."

"He's been very effective in those positions, but he has stayed away from direct medical care, unlike his parents."

"As I said, not exactly an asset to the Quinn family name."

"No, sir. Not yet. But he has important connections or he wouldn't have gotten the chief DP position."

"Don't kid yourself. He only got that slot because of me. I could have easily shut him out.

But you know, Potek, there's always a reason for everything I do. And that's the only real connection that put him in that spot."

"Yes, sir."

"He'll need close monitoring, Potek. We've had four people in that job in less than two years. They all lacked the guts to make the hard decisions. Let's see if a Quinn has the balls to do what has to be done." He paused. "And the operative we've placed in his office, Seka Joraine, do you think she can really stay close to the man?"

"Yes. As we agreed after her interview, I think she'll be perfect for this kind of assignment."

"What's the methodology of entrapment?"

"Familiarization. Chemical enticement. The third stage starts immediately. Sex is a very effective information gathering technique," Potek said with pride.

"How well I know." He thought of his frequent illegal use of chemicals to entice uncooperative women he really wanted to have as sexual partners.

"Excuse me?"

"Never mind. You never gave me the particulars of her agreeing to come on board.

How'd you get her to go along with it?"

Potek sat taller, almost strutted even though he remained in his seat. "As you know, she was recruited from Organ Harvesting. Every doctor assigned to that division requests a transfer, usually to no avail. She jumped at the chance."

"Is there anything special I need to know?"

"Sir! I can't reveal an operative's confidential history."

"Damn it, Potek, I swear, one day I'm going to throw you out on your ass. When are you ever going to get it into that thick head of yours that your corporation works for *me*? You're quoting my own god dammed orders. He took a deep breath. "Tell me more about the operative. Or do I have to look it up myself?"

Potek hesitated, but finally said, "Doctor Seka Joraine worked in Vessel Recruitment—"

"You're really pushing my buttons today, Potek. I know all of that already. Tell me something I don't know."

"Joraine was an excellent retriever until her parents committed suicide a year ago. After that, her manager's assessments show a gradual decline in her work status. Her production had begun to bottom out."

"I see. Well it'll be interesting to see how well she does as

Quinn's executive assistant." "Yes, sir."

"Good! Very good, indeed."

"Thank you, sir. I know she's highly motivated."

"I hope so," Dutton said. "I'm beginning to lose confidence in human resolve. Let's see what a Quinn does with that position. But if the trend continues…well, maybe it won't be quite so bad if it's Nathan Quinn who goes down."

Dutton turned around in his custom-fitted chair and stared out the window again. "Keep a close eye on Dr. Quinn and his new assistant."

"They'll be under constant surveillance, sir. Both auditory and visual. She wouldn't dare foul up this one-time opportunity."

"Maybe. Regardless, I want her reporting directly to me, as we discussed."

"I understand."

"That's all for now, Potek."

Chapter 12

Cable Car Conglomerate
Corpmall #1

Zoe Hidalga considered herself strong-willed, but right now, all she wanted to do was turn tail and run. Only exhaustion and inertia kept her sitting in the shadow of the mall's twenty-foot Mercian fountain. Her gaze took in the sculpture, an abstraction of cable cars that used to climb the San Francorp hills. Squashed aluminum tracks circled the outer edges of a miniaturized cable car with an elongated bell that topped the piece. It rang at irregular intervals. Zoe loved the sound of the bell.

It was right here at this fountain that she and Elliot plopped down to rest between their wandering through the different stores. At that time, the sound of water gushing through the varied metal parts created a lyrical piece with its own rhythmic beat. She and Elliot people- watched, created different stories about various people; some were so wild and far-out that they might have been about humanoids on another planet.

After Laya was born, they took her with them, taking turns holding her on their laps. And the baby laughed at the different people who couldn't seem to resist stopping to smile and admire her.

She was so beautiful. So beautiful.

When everything changed. Elliot became ill.

Zoe's eyes filled with tears as she stared at the same string of stores lined up all around her. But the fountain was now dry, like so many around the city. One day they'd simply been turned off without explanation. Everyone talked about it for a while and then seemed to forget that they ever operated. She could still imagine the gush of water cascading over the metal, some even splashing onto the ledge where she sat. Maybe the soothing bubbling sounds would have silenced the pounding in her head, allowed her to get past her anger at her friend Andrew. At this moment, she despised him.

She knew the tall black man was staring at her. She could feel his presence.

Zoe turned to face him. His hands balled into fists, tucked at his sides as though only tremendous control kept him from swinging at someone. The man staring at her with the chiseled lines of tension in his face made her realize how the last two years had stolen away simple expectations of love, friendship, and loyalty.

And now, the final loss was Andrew. He'd betrayed her; he'd betrayed Elliot.

That thought alone left a gaping hole in the center of who and what she was.

It was a simple equation. He could have saved my husband, his friend. Could have saved the man I loved. But he didn't.

The Corpmall coffee shop's doors flew open and everything turned into a whirl of Corporit-coded colors as they gushed out like the spring rains she remembered as a child. The younger people were laughing, talking playfully, moving at a rapid pace. Older men and women walked with a more deliberate step. But everyone was focused on getting to their job. Even Zoe glanced at her watch. Being late wasn't an option if they wanted to stay employed in the Corporit system.

She couldn't stop thinking of Elliot. She remembered how she'd pleaded with him to seek medical assistance. He'd refused, said it wouldn't do any good. And Andrew had agreed it was unnecessary as long as he was there to help her.

Those weren't just empty words. Andrew had stayed, tended to everything including changing putrefied dressings. As the purple lesions grew in numbers, they began to fill with pus. The constant ooze required fresh dressings and Andrew helped Zoe not only with that rank smelling necessity, but with every single needed thing, even caring for Laya.

And he'd been there at the very end in that stark hospital room that smelled of disease and darkness, the place where she watched death crush, then snatch her husband away.

And with Elliot's death, Zoe's life had ended, too.

Everything shut down. All that remained was a numbness that never thawed. She refused food, didn't care for Laya. They medically diagnosed her as nonfunctional. Only Andrew's intervention had saved her from being chemically neutralized. With her past erased, not only would she never have seen her daughter again, she wouldn't have recognized her if she had.

Andrew saved her. But he didn't save Elliot, and he could have.

Why?

She stared at Andrew's familiar dark, rugged features and wanted to run from the mall, to get as far away from him as possible.

But there was no place to go. No home, no work, no husband, no daughter, and there was no energy or will for anything.

"Believe me, Zoe," he said, interrupting her thoughts. "I didn't just let Elliot die. I did all I could for him at the time."

"If only I could believe you."

"You have to. You're not going to make it without me. We have to get away from this spot. The longer we stay here arguing, the greater the danger to both of us."

His voice sounded muffled, then far away. Her world tipped into a slow spin as her eyes lost focus, knees turned to water. Andrew lifted her, steadied, half-walked, half-carried her toward the nearest transit tube.

"Andrew, I can't fight anymore. I feel so weak. So tired."

"You just need some rest."

He propped her against a wall, held her in his arms as though they were lovers, then casually removed his telelink and tapped in a number.

"Tia, it's me, Andrew." He waited a beat.

"I know I'm late but it's unavoidable."

Zoe listened to Andrew. He was trying to remain calm, but she could tell he was in some kind of trouble.

"Listen carefully. You'll have to start the new model seventeen jay-jay presentation without me. You're as up to speed on the process as I am."

Andrew paused and Zoe heard a raised voice on the other end of the telelink.

"Stop stating the obvious," Andrew said "We both know they're not going to like it. But that doesn't mean they won't buy the concept when they hear about it from you. I chose you to work with me, Tia, because of your robotic training. You're as good a technician as I am. And you know it. You can do this."

Zoe studied his face. Lines she'd never noticed deepened as he spoke.

"I still need you to do it." Andrew's voice was tense and demanding. "Stop calling me Dr. Potter. I know you're upset and I don't blame you. I'd be there if I could."

He waited a beat, wiping the bubbles of sweat from his brow.

"I owe you. Thanks, Tia."

Zoe watched Andrew tuck the telelink back into his pocket and scan the area again. The mall was virtually empty now. Most Corporits were back at their jobs, settled in for the day; it was still too early for the shoppers to wander in.

He waited a few moments, gave Zoe a reassuring smile. Again, he made sure no one was following as he held her, then walked them toward the entrance to the electro-magno express pod entrance.

Everything around them became unfocused, a watery smear. She tried to hang onto consciousness but it was drifting away.

"One foot in front of the other. That's all you have to think about, Zoe."

"I'm so tired, Andrew."

Her feet felt strange as they stepped on an ambulated belt. It carried them down to the pod area. From far away, she watched Andrew insert his Ident-card and punch in a double fare.

Chapter 13

Medi-Prog Complex
Conference Room A

Nathan Quinn glanced at the conference table, a solid hunk of white plastin that, along with the chalk-white walls, made all the Medi-Prog chiefs appear as if tossed together into a large empty box. Or was it a fish bowl?

He scanned the faces of the others. Their eyes were dull with boredom.

Who could blame them? It wouldn't surprise him if someone was watching him and thinking the same thing.

Boring!

Emory Dutton droned on and on, not only about the Corporit medical structure and its selfless service to society, but also about how Corporit life was exciting and truly the ultimate human experience. Nathan had been in one or another statistical division of Corporit since he'd completed medical school and his internship. But the meetings were virtually all the same.

Every single meeting talks about the same crap.

After ten long minutes, Dutton finally turned the meeting over to the various Medi-Prog chiefs so the big man could judge their departments and their operations.

More boring, useless, drivel.

Nathan leaned back in his chair, tilted his head toward the head honcho of the Infectious Disease Department, who was now speaking. He remembered when his father held that position.

Most of the treatments and stats concerned VMAS. Nathan already knew a considerable amount about that particular disease.

VMAS had been dinner table conversation during most of his formative years when his father had been the chief of

Infectious Diseases. Now, the elder Quinn was an unhappy consultant to the unit. Only when pressed would he admit his satisfaction—and luck—with being able to continue working with the department once he reached the Corporit age limit of sixty.

But the Quinn family, with its longtime wealth and political influence, had an advantageous edge that many others could never dream of achieving.

Nathan fingered the multiple buttons on his mobile Doculslate, but instead of notes concerning the ongoing recitations, the screen showed nothing but a mess of scribbling, doodles, and sardonic questions. Most of what he'd written made no sense at all. He merely used the Doculslate as a prop, as if he was an actor in a play and needed to make it appear that his attendance was integral to the proceedings.

To think I bartered the Quinn name shamelessly ... schemed, plotted, and used every conceivable trick, to increase my odds of becoming one of these Medi-Prog chiefs.

And, to his surprise, it had worked.

He sat at this very table, this closed session, because now he *was* the chief in charge of Desisto Processing for Medicorp. He'd propelled himself into what was probably not only the top rung of his career ladder, but also made him an integral part of Dutton's elite circle that controlled medical care for everyone within an area once known as California, Nevada, and Arizona.

After Nathan had gotten the position, he finally told his father, who reacted unexpectedly.

"You've put yourself into a dangerous environment."

"I don't think so, Dad. Anyway, it was time for a change. Something more exciting."

"Well, just be careful. For god's sakes, stay clear of Emory Dutton…or at least stay on his good side. He hates our family."

"Why?" Nathan had been surprised. He'd never heard his parents mention Emory Dutton.

"I really don't know why. Years ago, we argued intensely over the dispensation of medical care. But in the end, things went his way. I thought that was the end of it."

"So?"

"That man holds lifetime grudges. Anyway, the word is…he hates our family."

"But he must have been the one who gave the okay for my new job."

Nathan could still hear his father: "And he had some reason for doing that. Someday we'll find out why…trust me…we won't like whatever that reason is. You should have consulted with me first before you put yourself in that man's hands. Emory Dutton is despicable and has no conscience."

"But it's a great job, and at least I'm in a key position in Medi-Prog now."

Why wasn't Nathan in the throes of ecstasy? He'd gotten what he wanted. Life should be damn good.

Except everything has become way too complicated.

He never dreamed that he would end up involved with this kind of medicine. The more he researched the statistical background of the DP program, the more the human loss disturbed him; large numbers of people were being forcefully eliminated.

Murdered.

Zoe Hidalga was not some random statistic, nor were the other DPs. All of them were real people—sick, yes—but still people with hopes, dreams.

Just the name Desisto annoyed him. Desist—to stop, to cease. That's what it really meant. Tagging an "o" on the end was some strange maneuver to lead people away from the word death. Whom did Dutton think he was fooling? Everyone in the medical corporation must know exactly what it meant. When he looked at Emory Dutton's steely eyes, he realized the name had probably been his idea. It smacked of the CEO's warped reasoning.

Nathan finally accepted that he'd been naïve. That was the undercurrent of what his father had said…and he'd been right.

Dutton cut into the Infectious Disease report when the

Medi-Prog chief complained of recent staff reductions.

"Doctor," Dutton said. "I can see you don't like our quota system." There was applause from a couple of people, but it faded very quickly.

"Frankly," Dutton said. "I'm not too sure I would like being told where I could study and work either. But quota control is absolutely essential. Remember, at the turn of the century the competition for patient and government dollars made too many people leave the medical profession. Now, without government interference, corporations can do what is necessary. We know and respect the value of the dollar. Besides, it guarantees you a well-paid job." There was a light buzz of conversation until Dutton tapped the rim of his water glass with a metal straw.

"Back to you, Doctor." Dutton pointed a finger at the chief of Infectious Disease. "Your staff is more than adequate. However, we want you to be happy. We will reduce *your* compensation by half. Then we can fund another professional. Will that be satisfactory?"

The MD gave a negative shake of the head.

"I didn't think so."

The chief of Infectious Control looked down, his face had blanched and he was breathing hard.

The CEO walked the length of the conference table before returning to his seat. With a sweep of a hand, he included all the doctors at the table. "You're all too independent, too resistant, and most of you still imagine yourselves as healers. Well, let me tell the healers in the room that we're not short of physicians now. Why? Because *we* control the numbers. Corporate management works."

Dutton stopped; a smug smile crossed his face. For some reason he was looking at Nathan's brand new assistant, Seka Joraine. She sat along the outer edge of the conference table with the other chiefs' assistants. Nathan watched her stare back at Dutton for an instant before returning to her Doculslate.

Nathan swallowed hard against the tightness in his throat. He shifted in his seat to release the built-up tension. Even though

Nathan's father had warned him about Dutton, Nathan had now reached the same conclusions on his own.

There was something malicious about Dutton. Each time the CEO spouted corporate propaganda about the medical system, Nathan wondered why years ago he had fought so hard to be among the privileged few who were accepted each year for medical training. He'd had his choice of any corporate program. After all, with his name he could have picked any field to follow. But Nathan chose medicine, as his parents had.

But for many years now, he'd been more of a businessman than a healer, even with the MD designation after his name.

Dutton's voice became a distant buzz.

Reality struck hard when, during his medical training, Nathan discovered that in the future he wouldn't have direct contact with patients. His parents had tried very hard to steer him away from medicine in the first place, tried to warn him that he was too idealistic for the state of the profession.

Why let the facts get in the way of what I wanted?

Still, reality hit him hard. As predicted, he never once touched a sick person after his internship; the closest he came physically to anyone who needed his skills was with his activated treatment plans, programmed daily into hospital computers. No doubt, it was the most economical, efficient way to manage large numbers of patients with minimal staff, but he hated it.

"…Desisto Processing doing?"

It took Nathan a moment to separate reverie from the present. He looked up; everyone stared back at him.

He pressed the buttons on his Doculate; his heart hammered against his chest. He'd almost been caught with his pants down. He had no idea what Dutton was asking of him.

He gambled.

"Quarterly stats indicate the DP projections are right on target" He glanced briefly at the others; their eyes were still on him. It was obvious they were simply tolerating him and his report—with one exception.

Emory Dutton.

Dutton tapped a staccato beat on the table with his middle finger. “Go on, Quinn,” the CEO said. “It’s getting late.”

Nathan checked his anger. He didn’t even like being in the same room with Dutton. He shifted in his chair, knew his face had turned a bright red, cueing Dutton that he hadn’t been paying attention. He probed his memory while he pretended to read from the scribbles on the Docuslate in front of him.

“In the past three months, DP has sanctioned five hundred elders, five hundred and sixty- two afflicted, and eleven hundred and forty Defys. This, of course, is strictly from among the Corporit population.”

“And the Noncorps and Aughts?” demanded the CEO.

“I can give you figures for the Noncorps. CARE units keep close track of them…at least for those who use that system. But the Aughts are much harder to nail down; they’re nomadic and uncooperative.”

“It’s your job to bring me the answers, Dr. Quinn.”

He tried to recall the Noncorp statistics he’d seen the day before, tried to visualize the numbers.

“The numbers for the older population are significant, even though they’re only a small percentage of the Noncorps,” he said, stalling. “Most elders are not willing to leave the safety of Corporit structure.”

“Yes, yes! We know all of that, doctor. What are the actual numbers?”

And there, in his mind’s eye, the figures appeared out of nowhere. He inhaled deeply and said, “CARE has sanctioned two hundred and sixteen elders and fifteen hundred and ninety-five afflicted.”

Dutton nodded curtly. “I want solid Aught data, Dr. Quinn.”

“As you know I’ve just taken this position,” Nathan said. “It’s going to take some time to get up to speed.”

“That kind of response doesn’t fly here, Dr. Quinn. Do your job! We need specifics and we need them on time.”

Dutton looked out at the others.

"Are there any questions on today's reports or my comments?" When no one responded, he adjourned the meeting.

Nathan left the table; in the hallway, he quickened his pace until he caught up with Seka. "How was that for a wake-up call," Nathan said, walking beside his assistant.

"Just part of the job."

"I guess you're right, but I hate early morning meetings," Nathan said, smiling at her. "Not to change the subject, but we haven't had much of a chance to talk, Seka, since you joined the staff."

"Is there something in particular you want to know?"

"Not really. It's just that I like to know a little something about the people I work with. For instance, where were you last assigned?"

"I think that information is my file," she said. "However, I was an organ harvester in the Vessel Retrieval Division. " They moved onto the central ambulated walkway that circulated throughout the huge medical complex, connecting all the various departments.

"That must have been difficult work. I can't imagine what it must be like working on deceased children."

"I'd just as soon not talk about it, Doctor, if you don't mind." She gently touched his arm. "How long have you been a Medi-Prog chief?"

Nathan's arm tingled at her touch. He turned and looked at her, noticing her soft brown eyes for the first time. He also caught the faintest whiff of her perfume, combined with what could only be described as animal musk.

His groin stirred.

"You know, we could talk about this over dinner," Nathan said. "How about tonight?"

"I'd love to." As they reached the office door, she added, "Why don't I cook at my place?"

"Sounds quite nice. Can I bring something?"

"Just yourself."

She smiled as they entered the office.

Nathan was confused by the sudden turn their conversation had taken.

Chapter 14

San Francorp
Defy Safe House

Zoe drifted in space, her long black hair fanning across her shoulders to cover her nakedness. She was well, strong. And there was no sign of VMAS.

The air was sweet and held promise. A promise of what? She didn't know. But she sensed something was there waiting for her.

Floating, floating, floating in the softness of the unreal. An observer in a dream. Yes, this was a dream.

It would be dawn soon, but night shadows were still there, deep and mysterious—a backdrop to the flickering stars above her.

Ahead was an opening to a narrow corridor. She floated toward it, her body tugged along by an undertow until she reached a dissection lab. She recognized the place, knew exactly what building she was in—the place where she'd spent every working day since graduating medical school.

No, she wouldn't, couldn't go there. She pulled back, floated away again.

The stars were far away, but the land was near and growing nearer. She anchored a foot on the ground and the rest of her followed until she landed with a thump, settling onto a solid ledge on a mountain. Standing, she searched in every direction.

Nothing.

She was alone.

When she dared to look down, there was only a black void, but the sun was rising. Rays of golden light began to penetrate the vast emptiness.

A figure rose from the darkness below; a man. He floated up toward her, saying something she couldn't hear. Yes, now she could hear him.

"Zoe."

Rays of the sun glowed on his skin; he radiated a golden light. He moved closer, his arms open, reaching out. His amber eyes mesmerized, held her.

"Take a step, Zoe."

She didn't know this man, yet, she wanted to go to him, wanted to believe in him.

She held back, searched his intense eyes for answers she needed before she could surrender. But his words filled her head.

Take a step.

This being, this man, was beautiful, strong; he offered strength, reassurance, hope. She looked into his eyes and stepped into the void.

* * *

Zoe's eyes snapped opened, her breath came fast and hard. She was lost between the dream and reality. Her aching hands formed into reaching claws.

Her head was still foggy. She had no idea where she was other than in what seemed to be a large and very comfortable bed. She was suddenly filled with the rush of conflicting feelings that made her feel strange, lonely, fearful. Yet somehow, a heavy burden had been lifted. She felt an unbelievable sense of freedom.

She laughed out loud.

Oh, yes! I'm a free, crazy person...dying of VMAS.

Closed blinds shrouded the room, hiding details, furnishings in gray shadows. Zoe thought back; the last thing she remembered was talking to Andrew. She must have passed out in mid-conversation with him.

She tugged at one of several pillows and dragged it down under the covers until it was flat against her gut; it didn't ease her physical pain or the aching thoughts of her daughter.

"Laya," she murmured. "Will I ever see you again?"

Waves of chills made her tremble, forced her deeper into the bed. She tightened the covers around her.

Elliot, I'm so tired. Tired of living. Surviving is too much.

Too many details to think about. So much to do.

Her gaze was drawn across the room to a large painting. Even in the diminished light, she recognized it as an Arina Marek. Bright cadmiums screamed at her, tried to tell her something.

Elliot's face, his eyes, piercing yet unbelievably kind, rose up and out of the painting. As quickly as he appeared, he vanished between the impasto layers of pigment.

"Don't go," she whispered. She searched, probed every color, every nuance. But Elliot had vanished, lost in the reds and yellows. Then the blunt colors detached and hung free from the canvas like a hologram.

She squeezed her eyes shut to make the hallucination disappear.

When she dared to look again, the room had turned from a shadowy gray to the inky black of the universe. The pigment from the painting flew into free form, spinning into a huge image of someone else. This man had an ethereal glow surrounding his body. He shone in the darkness, shone an eerie light that illuminated every corner of the room.

He was the man from her dream. The Indian who had reached out to her.

How did she know he was an Indian?

She just knew.

He carried panpipes, which he began to play. Throaty, primal music spanned the distance between the two of them; the notes coiled around her body, leaving behind a flash of ecstasy that twisted and covered every inch of her skin. She knew she was lying down in a room, yet, as she stared upward, a starry sky blinked above in an unfolding universe.

A healing universe.

She saw nothing, yet she saw everything. Knew nothing, yet knew everything. No longer alone, there were arms to hold her, lift her, open her heart to everything that was or would be.

She was strangely reassured, yet disconnected at the same time. A thrilling chill crawled up her spine as the man moved closer.

So strange, so beautiful.

Zoe wanted to touch him, to feel his golden skin. But the universe receded and the painting's bold images reformed. The Indian was snatched, swirled into a wind-torn storm. Out of the confusion of color, a pair of penetrating amber eyes stared back at her. And she heard an unfamiliar voice.

"You can survive, Zoe," the image said. "You can! Just take the first step."

This is not real; I'm hearing voices.

But she knew that he *was* there. She could feel him inside of her, filling her with his words.

"You can survive."

"How can you know that?"

The hypnotic eyes pierced hers. "Believe! Envision a different future."

"I'm dying!"

"You can live. Surrender! Take the first step."

Zoe rubbed hard at her eyes. The features of the man's face were now etched with more detail. Craggy, weather-beaten. With a swirl of motion, the pigments reached out for her; she was tangled within its prismatic swirl. Her head spun. She closed her eyes.

Down, down. She slid down.

Strong arms caught her. Amber eyes floated at her side.

"I'm afraid."

"You will find your way."

Her heart pounded so hard she could barely breathe. She opened her eyes, reached out to touch the man. But he had dissipated, was gone.

Zoe pushed a comforter away, sat up slowly, and ran her hands gently up and down her sides. Cautiously, she slipped from the bed and walked unsteadily across the large room. She flipped the light switch and stared at the Marek painting.

Reaching out, she trailed shaking fingertips across the textures of the canvas. There was an energy there; she willed herself to absorb what was trapped inside.

"Take the first step," she murmured. She stared into the depths of the amber eyes, pressed a hand against her belly, doubting yet wanting to believe.

"What kind of future can I have with VMAS?"

Her voice trailed off, her mouth remained open.

The pain in her belly was gone.

* * *

When Zoe stepped out of the luxurious marble shower stall, Andrew Potter was standing in the bathroom doorway, his head turned away.

"Did you bring me here? Are you responsible for all of this?"

"Yes and yes," he said.

"Last thing I remember is the mall; we were having a conversation. Next thing I know, I'm waking up in that magnificent bed over there."

"You sort of lost it as we were getting on the e-m express."

She tried to remember, couldn't. But the vision she'd had as she woke up was still vivid in her memory. She wondered whether to tell Andrew about it.

"Tell me when it's safe to look."

She laughed. "You can look anytime. There's not much to see."

"You sound like you're feeling better."

"I did get a little rest," she said. "And a long shower helped. I've needed one since early this morning. How do you get away with not having a water meter?" She wrapped herself tightly in a blue bath sheet, let it absorb the moisture. "Okay, I'm decent now."

"It's time to leave the city," Andrew said after turning around to study her. "Yes, you definitely look a lot better."

"Leave now?"

"As soon as you can get dressed."

"What about Laya? I can't leave without her."

He reached out and rubbed a knuckle lightly against her

cheek. "One step at a time, Zoe."

"That's not good enough. I want my daughter with me."

"I'm working on that."

"Do you think I can just sit around hoping it's going to work out, trusting that someone else will do what I should be doing? I made that mistake once."

"You weren't responsible for them taking Laya away. You were half out of your mind with grief at the time."

"No! That's a rationalization I can no longer accept. I've relived that day time and time again. I did fall apart. They said I wasn't a fit mother and I let them take her. I couldn't let go of Elliot, and I couldn't hold onto Laya."

"It was a difficult time."

"Maybe, but I'm never going to let it happen again. I'm going after her."

"Zoe, don't be an idiot. You need to disappear…right now. If the CAPOs spot you, you'll never see Laya again."

"There has to be another way."

"And there will be. I promise."

She wanted to scream at him, beg him to get her daughter. But in the end, she crumpled into his arms.

* * *

"Where are we, exactly, and whose place is this?" Zoe asked. She was dressed and ready to leave, but Andrew handed her a steaming cup of tea and a piece of warm, buttered toast.

"You're safe here. Does it matter who owns it?"

"I guess not, but I would like to know."

"It's a place the Defys use, a safe house."

"Oh!" She took a bite of the toast, a sip from the cup, and gave Andrew a questioning look. "Butter? Green tea?"

"I have a secret source."

"How many other secrets do you have, Andrew?"

She leaned back into a sleek faux leather sofa, continued to sip the tea and nibble at the toast as she looked around the spacious room. Directly across from her were two chairs. The wide armrests and extended transparent lucine legs reminded her of a classic design used in the early twenty-first century. Purple cushions filled the chair's seat in a sharp flat spread of color that made the whole unit appear to float. She'd only seen pictures of these in her network. Being in the same room with them allowed her to experience just how truly remarkable they were.

The room had an array of photographs of an earth that had disappeared—waterfalls, forests, birds, animals, insects. But her eyes always returned to the opposite wall, to the huge oil painting of the nude Indian male. Earlier, when she'd stood before this painting, it had not only dominated the room, it had seemed eerily different. Or had she been dreaming? Had it all been a fantasy?

* * *

Andrew sat down beside her. "You have to understand, there was no way I could have helped Elliot. I didn't know about the VMAS stabilizer then."

She knew he was telling the truth; his eyes were steady and unwavering.

"No one knew it existed," Andrew said, "outside of an inner circle at the very top of the Corporit structure."

"How could that have happened?"

"Without a central government, all communications are under Corporit control. People are forced to accept propaganda as fact. No one knows what's really going on."

"But so many are dying, Andrew."

"And they're going to keep dying because the subterfuge is extensive and runs much deeper."

Zoe covered her face. "The CARE units are mal-programmed, aren't they?" she whispered.

"Yes."

"Bastards! They're allowing VMAS patients to suffer."

Andrew stood, walked across the room, and settled into one of the chairs again. "It's worse than that, Zoe. People are being deliberately killed. And not only VMAS victims. It's happening with all terminal diseases, to anyone with a chronic, long-term illness that requires extensive and expensive treatment. They may call it mercy killing or passive euthanasia, but it's really murder."

She looked into Andrew's eyes, tried to come to terms with a world that she never dreamed could exist. "And if I'd gone to a Corporit health counselor instead of the CARE unit?"

He looked away. "We wouldn't be having this conversation, Zoe. You'd be dead. Euthanized efficiently and economically, secretly neutralized under the Desisto Processing sanction."

"Elliot? Is that why you wouldn't let me take him to a hospital until the very end?"

"Exactly."

She stared into her teacup. "Why do they bother? No VMAS patient ever survives anyway. Wait a few months and it's over."

"Not orderly enough; not cost-effective," Andrew said. "Those few months use up many resources … and resources, as we're all painfully aware, are limited."

Zoe levered herself out of the sofa and walked unsteadily toward the door.

"Where do you think you're going?"

"I can't leave the city, Andrew. I have to get Laya first."

"Believe me, Zoe, you can't go out there; they're looking for you."

"I—"

"You won't survive. They have erased all of your accounts by now; no electro-mag travel, no telecommunications, no food credits. Nothing!"

Andrew moved to her side, wrapped her in his arms, whispered in her ear. "Nothing's changed. Getting your daughter will take careful planning. You go near her school and the CAPOs will pick you up on sight. Did you think they would forget about Laya? That's the first place they'll look for you. Probably waiting right now for you to show up. If not, the school principal will call them."

"But—"

"I know how you must feel, Zoe, but if anything, Corporit administrators are an orderly bunch. You're a glitch, nothing more than unfinished business that has to be settled as quickly as possible. And they won't stop until you're caught and sanctioned."

Chapter 15

Cable Car Conglomerate
Corporit Singles Complex #3

Nathan stood outside Seka's apartment door. His palms were slick with sweat. He clutched a dozen burgundy repli-roses in one hand, held onto a bottle of a rare white wine with the other.

He couldn't remember ever being this nervous before a date. The rush of excitement about seeing Seka was thrilling, but puzzling. He wasn't an impulsive person or someone who lost himself in instant passion. He chose his friends and lovers with care. If anything, he was overly cautious about his relationships.

What was the matter with him? He'd just met this woman. Besides, they worked together.

This wasn't a good idea, but here he was.

He juggled his gifts to reach for the doorbell, almost losing the wine in the process.

"Shit!" he mumbled as the door opened right away. He knew he must look like an idiot, fumbling to get it all together.

"Hi! Come on in!" Seka said, taking his arm. She eyed the flowers and wine with obvious appreciation.

He caught a whiff of her perfume; its effect was unsettling. It sort of reminded him of cut grass. Something he hadn't thought about in many years.

"Is that a bottle of Dobb's Chamaneau?" she said as he handed her the wine.

He could only smile; he was at a loss for words.

What is that aroma? Musk?

For some weird reason, her scent made him think of mushrooms.

"My God, how wonderful!" Seka flushed with excitement. "It's almost impossible to find this on the open market."

Nathan kept smiling but was disoriented. His crotch itched with hot sweat and a sudden ache burrowed into his groin. Why this sudden lust when he'd barely even thought about her until after the Medi-Prog meeting? Before then, the only thing they'd talked about was work.

He stared at her dress—an expensive Pegette original he'd seen one night when his holograph receiver tapped into the Nicole Fashion Channel. From the waist down, she was swathed in a frothy, shimmering pink that made him think of cotton candy. The burgundy, satin belt cinching her tiny waist was a perfect match for the repli-roses, creating a bold contrast to her filmy, white, see-through blouse. He couldn't believe this was the same woman he'd seen in his office wearing everyday go-to-work clothes.

Seka slipped the bouquet of repli-roses from his grasp as he continued to stare at her dress. With every breath, her breasts appeared and disappeared in the folds of the diaphanous blouse.

He suddenly blurted out, "You're beautiful, Seka." The intensity of his feelings jolted him.

"And you're sweet." She brushed her lips across his cheek and motioned proudly toward a matched pair of facing sofas. "Please, sit down! I just moved into this apartment this afternoon. Those sofas are brand new."

Nathan nodded. "Very nice."

"Excuse me, I'll be right back. I have the perfect vase for these flowers…and I'll bring glasses for this magnificent wine."

Her scent continued to wrap itself around him. Heavy, pungent; a combination of woman and earth.

Earth! How long had it been since he'd enjoyed the smell of real earth?

* * *

Nathan thought back to when he was just a little kid, off on a camping trip with his father.

Most of these outings were with the family, even though each year it took longer and longer to reach the tall trees and flower-filled meadows.

This was to be his last outing alone with his father, although he didn't know that at the time. It was weird—his father, who was usually a quiet man unless he was talking about medicine, talked nonstop, telling Nathan about their family history and their community contributions, how much he loved being a doctor, details about his Medi-Prog position, and the numerous advantages it gave Nathan.

"Roll down your window, Nat!" his father shouted. "Look at those trees! Smell them!"

Nathan hesitated, but did as he was told. He lowered the darkly tinted glass, fearful that unfiltered UV rays would penetrate the car's interior, injuring their skin and eyes. Only when the trees shadowed the entire roadway was he able to relax and enjoy the view. Soon, the pavement ended and they were on a hard-packed dirt road that eventually became a leaf-strewn forest lane.

"Isn't this beautiful, son?" His father jumped from the car, circled a giant sequoia, and motioned for him to follow.

"Come on, Dad, let's set up camp first." He was puzzled by his father's behavior.

"We can do that later, Nat. Let's go for a hike while there's still plenty of daylight."

His father moved briskly ahead as they slid in and out of the shadows; the sharp snap of crunched twigs reminded him of the special effects of the Chelsean symphony his father liked to listen to.

Each step scattered dead leaves and loose pine needles, released musty, pungent aromas into the crisp autumn air.

Rounding a giant redwood, Nathan plowed full force into his father, who had stopped to stare up at the mottled sun filtering through the tight interwoven branches. He reached for Nathan's hand and squeezed, put a finger to his lips, then pointed ahead of them. A misty shaft of light captured a fawn and doe grazing peacefully. Their heads came up sharply, their eyes turned toward them. Sensing no danger, the deer returned to their grazing. Everything was hushed, yet at the same time, alive with the sounds of birds and the rustle of breeze-tossed leaves. He remembered that day in the forest, a study of rich umbers, muted greens, dancing lights, and tantalizing aromas.

Earth aromas.

* * *

"Such a vibrant color," Seka said, holding a vase filled with the repli-roses.

"I wish they were real," Nathan said, still caught up in his reminiscence, wondering what had sparked that particular moment with his father.

"They're beautiful, nevertheless." She placed the vase on an end table. "And the wine! How and where did you get it?"

"Anything's possible with enough money." He couldn't believe such inane words were spilling from his mouth.

"It was very thoughtful of you."

He stared at her, was confused. The lights played some kind of visual trick. She glowed with a luminescence that made her face glitter with a silvery satin patina that exaggerated her dark, exotic eyes. He wanted to pull her into his arms, feel her breasts mold against his chest, knew she would be soft, warm, exciting.

He felt drugged, but so alive and exquisitely alert. Her gaze probed his until he tingled.

When she left to get the wine glasses, his mind emptied of his past life. He took a deep breath, got up, and crossed the room to a rack of Docudiscs. He browsed through the titles, all of which had something to do with medicine—*Organ Harvesting for the Living,* by Jabrel Darkas, MD; *The Ethical Treatment and Use of Animal Organs*, by Aani Michlin, PHD.

"Required reading," Seka said, back again at his side.

"I don't know too much about this field of medicine. I just…" He was becoming disoriented again, couldn't track what he wanted to say. He only knew he had to have Seka close to him … much closer than she was now.

His legs started to give way.

"Nathan, are you all right?" She held onto his arm and led him back to the sofa.

The spinning sensation passed after he sat for a moment or

two; he couldn't tell how long it had been. He watched from some place far away, as she poured wine into a pair of long-stemmed crystal glasses. The Chamaneau's bouquet filled the room.

They toasted each other with a soft tinkle of crystal, sipped the wine, and kissed.

Chapter 16

Outskirts of Corporit Area

Andrew and Zoe edged farther and farther away from San Francorp. Zoe couldn't stop looking back over her shoulder at the city's shadowy, mushroom domes. They hovered over the city—huge, impersonal, disconnected. She willed herself to take in, soak up different aspects of the cityscape as it receded. But it was disappearing too rapidly. Soon it would all be gone.

Left behind.

She wanted time to think about her many memories, wanted to picture everything in her past—her life with Elliot, with their daughter Laya. The three of them together. She wanted to see it all clearly so it would be embedded in her brain forever, so she would never forget. But she knew the details would be lost in time, in disconnection. Life had moved on. Her husband died; her daughter was taken from her. All of her precious memories would be hidden behind gauzy curtains that she wouldn't be able to see through again.

Questions piled one on top of the other. She couldn't put them to rest.

What was Laya doing right now? Was she sleeping? Dreaming? It had been so long since she'd last seen her. The school only allowed Zoe visitation every three months. Each time when the two of them were forced to part, Zoe cried for days afterward. And now she was leaving Laya behind. Could she be sure she would see her again?

The moon's hazy light made the nighttime world seem fragmented with eerie, dark, amorphous shapes looming all around them. It was strange and disorienting and the stimulants made it even more bizarre.

They passed long tracts of deserted residences, some burned-out shells, others still structurally intact within moonlit moats of shattered glass—empty homes that stood like orphans waiting to be rescued. She sucked in a breath from her oxygen canister and continued to think about her daughter.

For four grueling hours, they crept through abandoned residential and business districts on the outskirts of the Corporit zone, dodging roving CAPO patrols that appeared out of nowhere. After a while, they didn't dare walk standing upright. Over and over, the two of them crouched, crawled, crouched.

"Andrew! Please! I have to stop."

"We can't. We have to keep going or be caught … by the CAPOs … or the Aughts."

Andrew half dragged her forward every time she tried to sit. And all the time she knew every single step was taking her farther and farther away from Laya. Only the primal fear of being eaten by the roaming, seldom-seen night scavengers kept her moving forward.

Just as she neared the point of total exhaustion, was ready to fall to the ground and await whatever fate might have in store for her, Andrew raised an arm and pointed ahead of them. She could see, off in the far distance, what appeared to be an unguarded area.

"We can cross there into the Noncorp sector," he said. "Everything is quiet up ahead, at least for now."

Although the border was in sight, the landscape in between was filled with tall, unstable piles of concrete rubble, crumbling brick, rusted-out cars, discarded tires, broken furniture, and a vast variety of other detritus from a world that no longer existed. The mountains of debris looked as if they could tumble at any moment to create an avalanche that could bury them alive.

Zoe lost her footing several times as they set out across the vast acreage of trash. If Andrew hadn't caught her with each misstep, she would have tumbled into pits of jagged, rusted scrap metal.

"Not the easiest way," Andrew said, flicking on his flash to guide them through fields of useless scrap, "but the safest route I know."

They were almost at the end of the rubbish when they heard

a rumble in the distance.

Zoe pointed. "Look!"

A large vehicle, headlights and spotlights poking out into the darkness, raced toward them, parallel to the electrified border fence. It was impossible to tell exactly how far away it was.

"They've spotted us," she sobbed.

Andrew grabbed her hand and started running for the fence. Once there, he dropped to his knees and used his bare hands to claw at the loose dirt beneath the bottom wire.

Zoe started digging alongside of him. "They're going to catch us," she cried out. "We'll never get through in time."

"Don't look at them, just keep digging! Faster! Faster! Faster!"

The lights became brighter and brighter, the spotlights almost blinding them. Pockmarks of dancing dirt appeared all around them. Then they heard large caliber gunshots.

"Now!" Andrew yelled, pointing to the trench they'd dug. Zoe squirmed under the electric fence, expecting to vaporize at any moment. As soon as Andrew was on the other side, they took off running.

The patrol kept firing, trying to intercept the zigzag course they were improvising. Sprays of dirt and debris hit their ankles and legs, but the bullets themselves kept missing.

"Got to move faster," Andrew yelled. But Zoe's legs refused to give her one more step. Andrew grabbed her and pulled, half dragged her through more waste and rubble until they reached the remains of a brick storefront. Putting it between them and the patrol, they sank to the ground, rested against the bullet and wind-protected side of a wall.

Zoe was gasping, gulping, coughing, trying to catch her breath.

"Why did you bring me here? I don't want this…I want to go back! I need to get my daughter."

Andrew jerked her around, grabbed an arm. She could feel him tremble with rage. "You just don't get it, do you?"

"Get what?"

"Laya's safe where she is. It's you we have to get out of San Francorp. *You* can't go back! Ever! They know every one of your friends, every single schoolmate, every lover you've ever had. Friend and foe, they'll check them out." He shook her arm and yelled, "You've been cut from the herd, Zoe. They mean to hunt you down and slaughter you."

"Stop screaming at me! You keep saying the same thing over and over. I don't want to hear it again."

He let go of her arm, shoved his hands under his arm pits. "Do you want a fire?" he asked.

Zoe, hunched down inside her Zynec suit, nodded.

"Okay, I'm not sure what I'll find to make one, but I'll give it a try."

"I thought we had to hurry," she said.

"We do, but you need a rest first."

Zoe looked at him. She wanted to thank him for saving her life, but doubts continued to plague her about leaving Laya behind.

"It's not that I don't believe you, Andrew. I saw them strip my apartment. But kill me? That's just not logical. Everything you've told me sounds like more Corporit propaganda. I don't believe them…I don't believe you."

"Why all the self-denial? Think about what's happening … think about Elliot."

"It's so hard—"

"Remember your Corporit history, Zoe. It started so innocently, simply offering euthanasia to those who wanted to die, for whatever reason. But we've moved way past that. It's evolved into a depopulation program, euthanizing those who are not cost effective to treat. Now, it's progressed into withholding medical treatment for Aughts, Noncorps, and, finally, uncooperative Corporits, or anyone who could be labeled a Defy. To *them,* it's all *very* logical."

"Andrew, I—"

"I know it hurts, but look at Elliot. He was in double jeopardy…a Defy with VMAS. He didn't stand a chance."

"Did they know he was a Defy?"

"All they had were suspicions."

"Why didn't they arrest you? You were Elliot's closest friend."

"They picked me up, all right. Then after they tortured me, electro-juiced my gonads, they let me go." He grimaced at the recollection. "If they didn't need my robots, my techno mumble-jumble, they might have been less gentle and more insistent."

"I still can't believe Elliot was a Defy. I would have known."

"For God's sake, Zoe! We all worked together; we were friends. You must have at least suspected he was involved in something anti-Corporit."

She pounded the ground. "Never!"

"I'm sorry, Zoe. I warned him against being overprotective. And he kept promising he would tell you."

"Elliot," she murmured, tears welling up in her eyes.

Andrew tried to take her hand, but she jerked back, scooted away from him. "What the hell were the two of you up to?"

"Trying to make some kind of a difference. Trying to make things better."

"Well, you didn't get very far, did you?" She swiped at the gush of tears with the back of her hand. "Elliot's dead, and you're out here with me in the middle of nowhere. Some difference you've made!"

Andrew scrambled toward her, clamped a hand over her mouth, and said, "S-sh."

Zoe tore his hand away from her face. She expected him to grab her again, but he hesitated, put a forefinger to his lips.

"Listen!" he whispered.

She heard it…the sound of feet scuffling, scattering the loose debris.

"Probably Aughts," Andrew said. "The gunfire must have drawn them." He peeked over the wall, whispered back over his shoulder, "Can't see any of them."

"Can we make a run for it?"

"It's too far and we sure as hell can't go back the way we came."

"How far away are we from where you're taking me?"

"It's at least another hour to Asher Wind Storm's compound."

A rock flew over the wall and smashed into Zoe's arm.

She bit back a yelp. "We'd better do something, and quickly," she said, briskly rubbing the wound.

"Are you okay?"

"Yes, I—"

Six scrawny Aughts, rags barely covering their dirty bodies, vaulted over the wall. They whisked clubs back and forth in the dim light. Andrew snatched up a rock, but before he could put it to use, two one of them clubbed him to the ground.

Zoe rushed to his side, screamed at the attackers, "Are you crazy? I'm sick."

"Are you crazy?" one of the Aughts mimicked. "Are you crazy-areyoucrazy-areyoucrazy," he continued in a singsong falsetto while a crooked smile exposed black stumps in his mouth.

"Andrew! Are you all right?" She turned away from the mimic.

"Areyouallright-areyouallright-areyouallright!

Andrew moaned, rubbed his damaged shoulder. "It's okay, I can make it."

"I'm pleased to hear that," one of the others cackled, spinning in closer. "Aren't you, boys? Now we can have more fun with this asshole." He jabbed at Andrew's side with a long, pointed stick. "On your feet!"

Zoe tried to help Andrew, but the mimic yanked her hair and swung her aside. She screamed as she landed heavily on a pile of rocks.

"Let me help you up, little lady." The mimic grabbed a hand, pulling her up tight against him. He smelled like rot and garbage; she wanted to vomit. He jammed his other hand between her legs.

"Stop it! Why won't you listen. I'm sick."

"Listen-listen-listen!" He spun her around to face his friends. They watched silently as he worried the snaps of her jumpsuit, then yanked it open.

"These Corp'its are pretty, but they ain't got no guts. Can't even take care of their women."

The others danced around them, laughing and pointing at Andrew, who was still kneeling on the ground.

The mimic nipped at her neck and popped open enough snaps in her pants to shove his fingers inside. She wiggled, tried to yank her hips away.

"Like that, do you?" He giggled, trying to give her a slobbery kiss on the mouth. "Good!

"Keep moving your ass, Corp'it lady, and I'll have my whole fist up there."

She sharp-twisted, sank her teeth deep into his neck. He roared in pain as her mouth filled with his blood.

Part 2

Chapter 17

Bordering San Francorp
Noncorp Sector

Asher Wind Storm stared at the luminous glow of the moon. He willed the clouds to part; the sky blossomed with stars that hung like silvery dancing lights. Beyond, farther into space, he sent Earth greetings to the dark universe filled with racing molecules that whispered promises of other worlds. Storm opened himself to the magical wonders of the night and felt the breeze sweep through his hair.

Tonight, he would surrender to the powers within the eternal Medicine Wheel.

Tonight, he would sit within one of Earth's most sacred spaces.

Tonight, he would empty his mind, meld with the healing forces of the universal Sacred Hoop.

All of Mother Earth was sacred, all life upon it was to be honored. He knew the Medicine Wheel was a physical emanation, a spiritual symbol of the lore of existence; it held the wisdom that lived forever in everyone from the day they were born. Storm was seated at its core, the heart of this powerful circle, surrounded by his closest companions. Here he fused with the golden light, the perfect physical manifestation of spiritual energy. Within this circle, he would gather the energies of all living spirits—from the trees, the stones, the moon, from every creature that existed. All were here with him, safe within a powerful place where they could radiate and enclose each other.

Each cell is a part of everything that exists. My heart is their heart. Their souls are my soul.

All are one.

The distant moon cast a shadowy glow. The cold air brushed his naked body and he knew he must rid himself of the Balanced Mind.

His Earth mind.

Logic destroyed the pathway to his soul's understanding. Beyond that restraint, all can open their hearts and become one with the universal, all-seeing Spirit.

He lifted his arms as an offering of surrender. Soon, the golden light spread throughout his core being. Its ancient secrets expanded deep within him.

Storm spoke softly but his words thundered in the air.

"Within this wheel of protection our energies unite to commune with Spirit, Self, Nature, and Creation."

A cloud of frozen dust whooshed up and formed a perfect halo that swirled around him. He watched a huge gray wolf, a pathfinder and healer, morph from the spinning force. The wolf bayed at the moon and squatted at Storm's side. Man and creature spirit flowed in harmony.

Matched amber eyes shifted to the horizon.

"I am Wind." His face turned to the east where the morning sun would rise, then turned to look at the moon. He bowed his head and scooped up a handful of the wasted earth. His mind turned inward.

I am filled with memories and visions beyond any explanation. I see the beginnings, the roiling seas, the fertile land, the air fresh and clean. I see Mother Earth vibrant and alive.

Mother Earth, our mother, dressed in thick green forests, her oceans filled with life. This is the wondrous world of the past, our rich heritage.

No longer seen, but never forgotten.

He scattered a furrow of depleted soil from the barren hillock where they sat. A warm gust of wind caught and altered the particles, dropping them rain-like into a large loamy circle. It surrounded him, the wolf, and a small core group of men and women.

Revivers of Earth.

Revivers.

"Earth, Fire, Wind, and Water," he chanted. "Breathe life

again."

He lifted a delicate panpipe and studied the instrument, laced with intricately woven reeds taken from the heart of the long vanished wetlands. Lifting it to his lips, he slid his tongue along its length, moistened the dry grasses.

A high-pitched song harmonized with the music of the flowing breezes as he played. The air vibrated with uncharted sounds. He knew it awakened memories in the Revivers, memories of a once bountiful earth. Other accompanying instruments and voices picked up the haunting strain until it swelled into a glorious crescendo, piercing the emptiness of the valleys.

Tears filled Asher Wind Storm's eyes as he gazed beyond the enclosed circle toward what he knew was sun-baked desolation that stretched between him and the cold, lifeless synthetic Corporit cityscape.

When the song ended, he stood and stretched his lean, muscular body and wrapped himself in a rare cotton robe. He faced the growing expanse of Noncorp Caplac domes that rose like a sea of gigantic bubbles floating on the reclaimed earth. Within this Medicine Wheel, this very place where he stood, one more of his biospheres would be placed to join the growing network of life-sustaining modules.

Bit by bit, patch by patch, the globally linked Revivers were reclaiming the earth, making it fertile again.

His tears dried and he was filled with hope. The group linked arms to return home.

When he reached his quarters, he was handed a coded message from Andrew Potter.

Chapter 18

Aught Encampment

Godan blinked away the wind-tossed cinders and ash from the campfire and scanned the surrounding territory like a predatory bird. At the edge of his domain, he could see the Corp'its' latest mountain of trash. Some of his followers had already dug out sleeping burrows within the new, steaming refuse, seeking its warmth. Others raked through the new trash to scavenge the moonlit dregs.

He smiled. Each new pile spread out his territory.

His territory. One he'd fought hard for only a year ago on his twenty-fourth birthday. The former leader had been strong, and it had been a fight to the finish. The asshole was buried in one of those far-away stacks with the rest of the dead ones. When the wind turned, he could smell all of them rotting away.

That fool never thought I could take him. Never thought a dwarf could do him in. Well I beat you, you asshole.

Bony children dressed in rags ran through the Aught campground. They all stayed far away from Godan. They knew better than to get too close; too many of them had been knocked head over heels after getting in his way. He didn't like kids. Too much trouble for the little they could do. He listened to their squeals and laughter as they romped over rancid piles of trash, played hide-and-seek, slipped in and out of the maze of tunnels lacing the mountainous mounds of garbage.

A commotion caught Godan's attention. A screaming woman clawed frantically at an older honeycomb of rubbish where someone was trapped. He blinked once and again, turned back to focus on the horizon. Let them dig their own way out. Godan didn't owe them anything.

He gave a grunt of dissatisfaction as a nearby Aught started to chant. "Hullabaloo-skidoo-achoo-parlez vous. Hullabaloo-skidoo-ach—"

"Shut your face, you asshole!" snarled another Aught, sticking his head out of a garbage cave. "I've been listening to you sing that filthy, rotten, stupid crap of a song for days. Shut the fuck up or I'm gonna wring your fuckin' neck!"

"Hey, pissface, I'll sing what I fuckin' well please. Put your mudface back in your own stinkin' hole, you—"

"Enough!" Godan boomed. He turned and pretended to move toward them, shaking his fist. Both men ducked back into their caves, neither wanting to become a bloodied victim of Godan's vicious temper. It was no secret that anyone who crossed him never got a second chance. And they damn well knew better than to call him a dwarf, either. Behind his back, well, okay, but don't get caught. Or else!

The two men stuck their heads out again. Godan still held them with eyes reflecting firelight in their black marble orbs. He ran a finger down his hawk-like nose and across his thin lips. When he was certain he could expect nothing further from the two, he gave them the finger and howled with laughter that turned into a phlegm-clogged cough that wouldn't stop. He hacked and hacked, spit out the plugs of foulness, covering the ground in front of him until he could breathe again. But the rattling in his chest didn't stop.

He sat down at his lookout post again, worried an irritating pustule on his pockmarked face. The painful pimples continued to erupt one after another, always reminding him of his taunting mother. She'd said it was the evil in him oozing out.

And then she'd mocked him one day, one time too many. Without a word, he'd reached out and crushed her neck. Her black, damning eyes never left him until they were lifeless and blank.

Godan pulled a metal rasp from the folds of his dragging, grease-smeared coat, and began to file the three remaining nails on his other hand. He paid no attention to the festering scars where the other two fingers had been lopped off in battle with Tabo and his rival clan. Instead, he kept his surviving nails long and dagger sharp, lethal as any knife.

A smile crossed his face as a small band of his men snaked through the mounds, pushing and shoving a pair of outsiders ahead of them. When they came into the firelight, Godan saw blood dripping from jagged rips in the black man's Zynec jumpsuit. Each time the woman reached to help, she was jerked away by her long hair.

Corp'its!

* * *

"Let go of me, you son-of-a-bitch, or I'll—"

"You'll what?" screamed the Aught who had been yanking Zoe's hair repeatedly since their capture. She planted her feet and refused to move. The Aught twisted her hair and shoved her to the ground. He sprawled on top of her, straddled her hips, and pinned her arms over her head.

Andrew lunged toward them and was greeted with a sharp stick jabbed into his thigh. "Back off, asshole, or I'll kill you here and now," the Aught shouted, holding the bloodied stick at Andrew's throat.

Zoe's eyes flicked from face to face as the Aughts crowded in around them. She clenched her teeth, tried to stop crying, but they poked their toothless, emaciated faces in hers and she wanted to vomit from the stink of rot.

"Let's see what she's got under that fancy outfit," the stick-wielding Aught yelled.

"Save the clothes for me!" a female voice called out.

But the Aught tore at Zoe's body suit until he exposed her breasts. He prodded both nipples with an index finger, screamed to the crowd, "Shit, she's no better than our scrawny bitches." He looked for the leader's nod before he tore more of her clothing.

The dwarf jumped off his platform, grabbed Zoe's attacker around the neck with one hand, and tossed him off to the side. With a grunt, he lowered himself, taking the other Aught's place. Two men stepped forward. One pinned Zoe's arms over her head, the other grabbed her ankles and spread them.

"Leave her alone!" Andrew shouted, pushing aside his

guard "She's sick, god dammit!" He dove for the man holding Zoe's arms, knocking him off balance.

She screamed, "No!"

The Aught stabbed Andrew with the sharp stick. It splintered as it smashed into his shoulder; ragged shards protruded from the open wound. Andrew slumped, eyes glazed over. Zoe lashed out at the dwarf, but he laughed and bounced up and down, crushing her pelvis into the ground.

The crowd screamed, "Take the fingers! Kill the Corp'its! Take the fingers! Kill the Corp'its!"

Their leader roared at the sky, shaking his fist, "Take the fingers! Kill the Corp'its!" Laughing, he ripped open the rest of Zoe's jumpsuit and pushed down the front of his tattered pants.

"But not before I get a piece of her."

* * *

High above the screeching crowd, wind-driven clouds darted across the sky in a frenzy, concealing, then revealing the moon. The strange rhythm of the clouds faltered and circled into a billowing mass. The cold wind grew harsher, icier.

A sudden rumbling thunder silenced the Aughts. One by one they looked to the sky, fell to their knees. The clouds had become a huge, glaring eye.

Godan stood above the woman, his pants at his knees. He looked up at the amber eye, angry at the intrusion, even angrier at his own uneasiness.

"You're not real," he raged, shaking both fists at the sky. The kneeling Aughts glanced with fear at both Godan and the thing in the sky. But their leader offered no explanations, did nothing to reassure them.

Godan returned his attention to the woman. A stinging sheet of sleet caught him full-face, knocking him down. He yanked up his pants and whipped his coat around him.

The crush of sleet had not touched the woman at his feet.

He shuffled to one side, closer to the crowd of surrounding Aughts. "Kill the Corp'its!" he ordered.

When no one moved, he bellowed, "Kill 'em, you

cowards!" A couple of men stepped forward, but were struck down by a shower of fist-sized hailstones. No one else moved.

Godan was freezing, but the pustules on his face were painful and hot. He snatched a spear away from one of his raiders. He would kill the Corp'rits himself. He'd only taken one step when he was engulfed in a swirl of wind that tore at him. Jagged rocks shredded his clothes, cut into his skin. Blood dripped from his eyes.

* * *

"Hurry, Daddy! The ducks must be hungry." Zoe clutched a brown paper bag full of stale bread. As she skipped along, tugging at her father, she slowed at the sight of a man, his hands filled with the strings of a rainbow bouquet of helium-filled balloons.

"Hey there, little girl; you with the long pretty curls. Would you like one of these?"

She stopped and stared at all the beautiful colors, "Ooh, the purple one! Can I have the purple one, Daddy?"

"Give my girl a purple balloon, please."

As they neared the water's edge, with Zoe holding her beautiful purple balloon, they passed a homeless man sunning himself on the bench. The man pointed at the small picnic basket her father carried. "Any extra food in your basket, sir?"

They stopped.

"Do we have anything extra, Zoe?"

"No, Daddy. We only have enough for our picnic."

"Are you sure?" He glanced at the bag of bread.

She pulled it up and clutched it to her chest. It was hers ... and the ducks'.

Her father gently squeezed her hand. His eyes told her there would be other days to feed the ducks. She slipped her hand from his and walked up to the dirty man.

"We have some bread, if you'd like to have it."

The man smiled, displaying a nearly toothless mouth. "Thanks, little lady." As he took the bag, he held onto her hand and kissed the back of it. Flustered, she let go of the balloon and it sailed up and away, until it was only a dark dot in the clear summer sky.

* * *

Zoe's eyes opened; a large gray wolf stood over her, its golden eyes within inches of her face. Before she could react, the wolf licked her cheek and looked away, panting softly. She raised her head. The animal stood between her and the crowd of Aughts. In the glow of the campfire's dancing flames, their faces were masks of confusion and terror.

Then she saw Andrew; his black face had turned a pasty gray. She crawled toward him; the wolf stayed close, moving with her.

The Aughts wavered, their circle broken; some disappeared into the darkness, others skittered back as the shadowy figure of a tall, muscular man entered the circle of light. The wolf's fur brushed against Zoe's skin as it trotted forward to stand by him.

Zoe's teeth chattered. She tried to pull the torn pieces of her jumpsuit across her. But the man moved closer and the air warmed around her.

He stopped and knelt over Andrew, floating his hands over the limp body from head to foot, stopping at the wounded shoulder. After a moment, he raised his head and nodded to Zoe.

His face was familiar. Yes, she knew this man. She looked from man to wolf and back again. The eyes. Amber eyes.

He was from her dream at the safe house.

The man stood, signaled to two companions. They lifted Andrew, settled him on a crude litter, and took him away. Then the man moved to her side, and in one motion, scooped her up into his arms.

Zoe watched the wolf pad around the fire's perimeter one last time. It came to a halt in front of the dwarf. The Aught leader wiped the still trickling blood from his eyes and aimed his spear at the panting animal. Before it could strike, the wolf vanished into the darkness.

Chapter 19

Hillsborough Mansionplex
Arina Marek's Quarters

Zoe was screaming, clawing at the face of the naked Aught who was crushing her throat. He pressed harder, harder, and when he relaxed for a moment, she scrambled out from under him and raced down through piles of trash in a blood-drenched landscape.

She covered her ears against the Aught's taunting laughter. She escaped, folding into a thick roiling fog of acid-laced vapor. The billowing poison spread through her lungs. She coughed, couldn't stop, coughing until she was spitting up blood all over everything.

Choking, lost, she clawed her way over massive boulders. Her hands were raw and bleeding. But she had to find her daughter so everything could be real again. Bursting into sudden light, she saw a girl skipping under a clear blue sky that glowed with radiant sunlight.

It was Laya skipping toward her; birds were everywhere, celebrating with trills and vocal arabesques. Then Laya looked confused, seemed to lose her way. She turned and drifted away.

The faster Zoe ran, the faster her daughter moved into the distance, flying over one filmy layer of light to another.

"Laya!"

Zoe bolted upright in bed, drenched in sweat. For a moment, the sounds of birds echoed in her mind. Then they were gone.

She was alone in an unfamiliar bed, in an unfamiliar room.

"No! Laya!"

Was it only a dream? Dreams and more dreams?

She fell back, clamped her eyes shut, pulled the covers over her head, held her fists tight against her gut. After a moment, she realized there was no pain. Nothing! And she felt different, stronger.

Zoe hugged herself, remembered how it had been in the past—warm and comfortable in bed, in Elliot's arms. Laya playing safely nearby.

Gone. All gone.

* * *

When Zoe finally opened her eyes again, a tall, broad-hipped woman was standing at the foot of the bed, backlit by sunlight that filtered in through a tint-safe window.

Zoe wiped at her eyes to clear her vision.

The woman moved to her side; streaks of bright purple highlighted her long hair. She looked down studied Zoe. Her eyes were warm and friendly.

"You're safe here, Zoe."

"Andrew? Where's Andrew?"

"He's alive, but—" Zoe sank back into the bed, expecting to hear the worst. "—he's not here. He's back in San Francorp."

"San Francorp? How is that possible? He was hurt … ripped apart," Zoe said, shivering, remembering every detail of the bloody scene at the Aught's camp.

"He did what he had to do. And he *had* to return to the city immediately."

"I don't understand…he lost so much blood…where did he find the strength?"

"Whatever was necessary was done for him."

Zoe ran her hands restlessly across the plump comforter and tossed it aside. "I have to go, too. I'm going back."

She started up from the bed, but the woman held her shoulders. "Didn't Andrew explain? You can never return to the city."

"But that's where my daughter is, where my life is."

"Stop wanting what you cannot have. Envision a different future, Zoe Hidalga."

She gazed into the woman's sea-green eyes, puzzled.

"That's what he said," she whispered.

"Who?"

"The man who carried me out of that horrible place. The man I saw in—" She couldn't bring herself to talk about her dream back at the safe house in San Francorp.

The woman sat down on the edge of the bed and took Zoe's hand.

"Storm's a wise man."

"Storm?"

"Yes, Asher Wind Storm. He's the one who brought you here."

Zoe looked around the large, bright room. "Here? Where am I?" She looked beyond the red and yellow quilt and the bright peach curtains draped around the window, thought of the place she'd called home until yesterday. This room radiated life; her apartment had been more like a cell, a tomb.

"Where am I?" she asked again.

The woman laughed warmly, tossing her purple-streaked hair off her shoulders.

"You're exactly where you're meant to be, Zoe," she said, standing up again.

"Stop it!" Zoe shouted. "Stop talking in riddles."

Envision a different future. You're where you're supposed to be.

"I'm not a child. I'm looking for answers, real answers." She pointed at the woman, "Who are *you*?"

The woman pressed her hands against her hips, light glinted on a large silver medallion hanging from her neck, its center was emblazoned with a replica of the stormy eyes that had frightened the Aughts.

"You're right! I should have introduced myself. I'm Arina Marek." Zoe stared at the woman, looked her up and down. "The artist?"

"Yes, I am an artist. This is my house."

Zoe's breath caught. "I know your work. Until yesterday, I owned two of your paintings," she said. "They meant so much to me."

"That's very kind of you, but Andrew told me you've lost a lot more than a couple of my paintings."

"Not lost. Taken!" Her hands balled into a fist. She stood and took a tentative step, would have fallen if Arina hadn't caught her.

Zoe covered her eyes and sobbed. Arina hugged her, ran soothing fingers through her hair, rocked her like a child.

Chapter 20

Hillsborough Mansionplex

"I burned that Zynec jumpsuit of yours," Arina said. "Even if you wanted to, there would be no way to piece it together. We need to find something else for you to wear."

Zoe had been sleeping on and off; now she crawled out of the bed and sat on the edge of the mattress. She needed a reason to get up and move because all she really wanted to do was burrow back in and hide her head under the covers, hide from reality and the decisions that had to be made.

She didn't want to think about what her tomorrows would be like in this alien Noncorp world, a world where CARE treatment centers lied, told her she was healthy when she was dying from VMAS. Lies. Is that what the Noncorps were all about?

Andrew might trust these people, but I don't.

But she was feeling stronger and more hopeful; that alone was reason enough for her to allow the artist to lead her across the spacious room to a closet that spread across a full wall. Zoe had never seen a closet this large, and when Arina slid the door open, it was jammed with garments of every description. The brilliantly colored clothes almost took her breath away.

"My God!" Zoe said, staring at a mélange of purple, yellow, green, red, and every possible variation of those colors.

"Hard to believe," Arina said. "Most of these clothes used to fit me." She touched several of the garments and smiled, then patted down her hips. "Take whatever you want, but don't even think of looking for any of those Corpmall monstrosities they call fashion. You won't find them here."

Zoe fingered the pieces of cloth. It had been a long time since she'd had any interest in what she put on her back. She pulled out several outfits, held them against her. She finally selected a red and blue paisley skirt and blouse combination and wiggled her way into it. When she stared at herself in Arina's full-length mirror, her excitement faded.

"Look at me!" She gathered, pulled, tried to deal with the material that hung around her as though she didn't exist.

"A few tucks here and there and you'll look beautiful," Arina said, reaching for her sewing kit.

Zoe looked in the mirror again, then sat down on the bed. "What am I going to do?"

"Stop it, Zoe!" Arina's voice was harsh. "Stop feeling sorry for yourself! Stand up! Get off that bed! Put one foot in front of the other, and at least take some responsibility for your own life."

"What are you talking about?" Zoe said, stunned. "Is it my fault my husband died? I would have done anything to keep him alive. And do you blame me for having VMAS?" She stared hard at Arina. "Responsibility? Hah!"

"You've been a doctor in the Corporit system all of these years. And did you ever question what was happening around you, question who was controlling your world? No! You went to work every day and never fought back. You followed the crowd, did what you were told."

"I had what I wanted: a husband, a child, a home. What's wrong with that?"

"Elliot knew the answer to that. That's why he became a Defy."

"What did Elliot see that I didn't?"

"He opened his eyes and saw it all. He risked his life to rebuild a free-thinking society."

"That was Elliot's choice. One he made without me."

"Can't you see? Corporits, Noncorps, all of us share the same world. And it's dying! The Revivers can't overcome the destruction of the planet without using every resource that's available. You need to become a resource, a human resource."

"The Revivers?"

Arina stared at Zoe, shook her head. "I can't believe how truly ignorant you are."

"Who are the Revivers?" Zoe said.

"Asher Wind Storm, the man who saved your life? His Revivers are a network of people around the globe. They're reseeding our planet. Elliot was a part of all of that, too."

"All *I* ever wanted was Elliot and Laya."

"Uh huh. And now you have neither. And the Corporits? They want you dead, Zoe. Can't you see, it's time to fight back? Take back your world."

"Look at these arms!" Zoe thrust them in front of Arina. "You know what these purple lesions are? I have VMAS. I'm going to die! Not much time to fight anything."

"Your disease doesn't have to be fatal. Andrew told you about the stabilizer."

"Look, I appreciate your help, Arina, and I certainly respect your talents, but I didn't ask to be here."

"You couldn't stay where you were."

"What's the difference? Stop treating me like an idiot. VMAS is fatal. Elliot died from it. So will I."

"You can survive. You have a chance, one that Elliot didn't have."

"How could you possibly understand what I'm going through?" She shivered, pulled the comforter from the bed, and wrapped it around her shoulders. "In twenty-four hours I've lost my home, my job, and worst of all, my child is left behind in one world and I'm in another. We might as well be on different planets. And you want me to believe in miracles?"

"I want you to fight back, Zoe. But all I hear from you is Corporit bullshit. You've been indoctrinated with Corporit mind sludge and it won't allow you to accept anything outside of those cloistered domes."

"You want me to be a believer?" Zoe said. "Get my daughter back! From where I sit, you and the Noncorps are just as helpless as I am."

"Give us some time, Zoe."

"Everyone talks about time as though that's all I have. Well, it's the one thing I don't have… time to spare."

Arina gathered up the clothes Zoe had tossed away and began to sew. She remained silent.

"Admit it! You're as much at the Corporits' mercy as I am," Zoe said. "You don't even know that the CARE units are lying, misdiagnosing, manipulating you."

"We know."

"We who?"

Arina hesitated. "Andrew, for one. And other people you can trust."

"Can they get Laya out of the city? Can they save my daughter?"

"When the time is right, it will happen."

"There's that impossible word again—time. Arina Marek, you may be a great artist, but I think you're an even greater liar."

* * *

Arina completed the alterations to Zoe Hidalga's clothes and decided to take her on a tour of the large house. She felt uncomfortable with her earlier curt behavior, knew she'd been hostile to Zoe.

What bothered her the most was that she knew she was taking out her hostilities toward the Corporits and their suppressive system on a woman who was ill, suffering, and needed her help. Arina knew she had a reputation as a person with little patience, but it was time to exhibit what patience she did have.

Zoe was obviously impressed with the size of the large, colorfully painted rooms. It was easy to understand—Arina was aware of what the average Corporit's apartment was like.

"Can you believe only one family occupied this huge mansion at the turn of century?

Hillsborough was quite the exclusive neighborhood for your Corporit forefathers."

"And now?"

"Like most of these old buildings, theyve been divided into several apartments so many people can live well."

The tour ended at Arina's studio. An assortment of partially painted canvases sat propped on easels awaiting her return. Interspersed throughout the room were unfinished sculptures in clay, stone, and metal. Several reached up to the twelve-foot ceiling.

Arina watched Zoe move from piece to piece, canvas to canvas, raw pleasure lighting her face. When she touched the sculptures, Arina could see the doctor trying to sense what was in the heart of the artist, in the heart of the creation. Zoe was really a true aficionado.

"I'd love for you to pose for me," Arina said. "In those exotic colors, you remind me of the women in classical Hispanic paintings."

Zoe looked pleased by Arina's request, and it was obvious that she was beginning to relax and really look at what was around her. She tugged at her blouse. "I've never once seen colors and patterns like this in the Corpmall."

Arina laughed. "Individuality has been bred out of the average consumer; blandness has become the Corporit norm."

"Have you always lived here?" Zoe asked. "With your talents and reputation you could live in San Francorp … or anywhere else you wanted to live."

"It was my choice to leave San Francorp."

"But why?" Zoe seemed truly at a loss to understand why anyone would want to leave Corporit willingly.

Arina was silent. She picked up a sprinkler can and began to the water plants that spilled out of every odd corner in the studio. She whistled softly to each of them as she made her rounds.

"Life is filled with inconsistencies," Arina said. "The greatest being that I never wanted to be an artist."

"But your works…they're fantastic." Zoe pointed at one canvas, then another. "Look at these women, their strong features, the bold colors. I want to know who they are. What they're thinking. What *you're* thinking."

Arina ignored her, hoping somehow the subject would roll over into something else. But she could feel Zoe's eyes demanding an answer.

"These paintings have been an outlet for my pain, my frustrations. That they gained recognition amazes me."

"I'm not sure I—"

"I'd never touched a paintbrush until I came here twenty years ago. I could just as easily turn my back on it now and never paint again."

"You can't mean that. You're so talented."

"Talent? My talent is no greater than yours."

"Don't be silly. I'm a doctor, and not a very useful one at that."

"Can't you hear yourself? A *doctor*! And in a world filled with the sick and dying."

"But anyone given the opportunity can study to become—"

"Zoe, tell me why a silent work of art moves us more than those suffering around us?" Arina turned away and ran her fingers down the length of a clay torso. "You probably don't know this, but I was a nurse when I lived in the city."

"I didn't know that."

"I refused to continue to take part in the Corporit depopulation programs."

"I've heard rumors about those programs. You helped with that?"

"Who else do you think hooks up the drugs that kill?" Doctors write the orders that are handed down from Corporit headquarters; nurses carry them out."

"Andrew said the same thing. But I can't get my head around it."

Arina couldn't stop herself, she spoke harshly as her temper flared out of control again. "You seem so dull-witted sometimes, Zoe! I still can't believe you were married to Elliot."

"For God's sake, Arina, please stop treating me like I'm some kind of backward child."

"Well, aren't you?"

"No, dammit, I'm not!"

Andrew was right. Zoe had really been kept in the dark

about Elliot's Defy involvement.

Arina circled the studio until she was calm again, then stopped to look out the window for several moments before she returned to Zoe and took her hands.

"There may have been a time when you could turn your back on the realities of Corporit tyranny, Zoe. That time is gone. Now, you're either with us or against us."

Chapter 21

Central Noncorp Sector

Zoe gave her cheek a final smear of protective skin lotion, adjusted her sunglasses and oxygen nasal tubing, and followed Arina out the door and down the steps of the mansion.

My parents were Corporits, I'm a Corporit, my daughter is a Corporit. I will not stay here...I will find my way home.

The artist had said very harsh things to her, but Zoe knew there was some truth in all of it. So she gave in and let Arina talk her into going out to see the Noncorp area. Zoe also knew she would need to learn everything, know everything about this Noncorp world if she was ever going to slip away and return to San Francorp to be with her daughter.

The light was ultra-bright even with her eye protection; her hands flew up to cover her face. When she finally was able to see again, she silently studied the landscape that surrounded several mansions that still remained in the area.

Fanning out from where she stood were numerous three-story, geodesic dome apartment complexes. Residential clusters were everywhere, spreading into the hills like a huge unfolding spiral.

"This is not what I expected."

"We have done so much," Arina said. "More than you can imagine. Everything we need is within easy reach of our homes—food, supplies, shopping areas are all pretty much in walking distance. And the open spaces? They belong to everyone."

Off in the distance, Zoe could see every open space hill covered with whirling windmills.

"Spectacular!"

"If you really want to see something beautiful, tomorrow I'll take you to the flat lands where the photovoltaic arrays are spread across the ground like a mosaic of mirrors. The light not only reflects the sun and helps us generate power; it covers up the ugly decimated earth and gives it real purpose."

Zoe had only heard the Corporit propaganda of how the Noncorps were failures at surviving. Yet, everything she saw in this world told a completely different story. Here, people were rebuilding, recreating a new society, all very much different from the closed off city that she'd just escaped from.

"Come on." Arina pulled Zoe farther down the street until they were in the middle of a crowd of laughing people, squealing children running in and out and around everyone. Most wore eyes medallions, like the one that hung around Arina's neck.

"Why do so many wear those neck pieces, like yours? Is it some kind of religion?" Arina stopped in her tracks and laughed until Zoe was not only annoyed, but perplexed.

"Well, I'm glad I can amuse you so easily."

Arina held out a hand, palm up. "No, no, no. I'm not laughing at you. I just haven't heard that question for a long time. She reached out and took Zoe's hand and smiled. "The eyes medallions are worn by the Revivers, the people who are followers of Asher Wind Storm's environmental rebirth system."

"Isn't every Noncorp part of that?"

"Not really. Not that they don't benefit from it," Arina said. "But many here are outcasts that have left Corporit for political reasons only. They form their own groups, follow their own interests. You have to understand, Zoe, this is an open society where many different voices and philosophies come together, live together in peace, whether they think alike or disagree."

"Isn't survival more important than anything?"

"There are some here who might even disagree with you about that," Arina said.

What a strange, complex world this is.

But the vitality of the Noncorps was such a dramatic contrast to the harsh realities of Zoe's Corporit lifestyle of separation, loneliness, and regimentation. It was difficult to absorb.

"It's so weird to spend so much time out in the open like

this," Zoe said. "I don't think I've seen such a large spread of the sky since I was a little girl."

"We don't spend a lot of time out here either unless we're geared up," Arina said. "Air scrubbers inside, oxygen nose cannulas outside. That is, if you want a pair of decent lungs in your chest. Or if you want to live past thirty."

"I guess the San Francorp domes have *some* value."

"Yes, they do. They keep you locked up."

* * *

"This is what doctors do in our world," Arina said to Zoe as she led her into a reclaimed brick building. Inside the reception area, the first thing Zoe noticed was all the walls were covered with large paintings. They were unmistakably Arina Marek's work—wild colors, abstractions of nudes.

The room itself was filled with people of all ages. Some were talking, some just sat quietly. Many were coughing and looked very ill.

"Those are your paintings, aren't they?"

"Ah, yes," Arina said with a big smile on her face. "I have to admit I love seeing them hanging on the walls in all their wicked splendor."

"They're incredible."

"This is one of our medical clinics, Zoe. There are many of these in the Noncorp world. They're divided throughout the communities as a vital part of the healthcare we try to provide."

"But I thought the CARE units—"

"The CARE units are helpful, but are only a small part of what's needed for our growing population."

"And hospitals?"

"We need more, but the ones we have are well staffed."

"Who treats the patients here?" Zoe asked, indicating those in the room.

Arina laughed. "Doctors and nurses, of course. If you lived in our world, you could become a real doctor again and give direct care to people who need you."

"I'm not sure I'd remember how to do that," Zoe said.

"You'd be surprised. Many doctors feel as you do when they first come here. But all medical personnel work together. They would help you find a way to put your skills to use."

* * *

When they left the building, Arina took them down a nearby side street. "And this is where I hang out when I'm not working."

Displays of art were everywhere; paintings and sculptures lined the sidewalks. Someone was playing a piccolo and the music gave the scene an added sense of movement and fun. Arina, in her coral blouse and orange and black flowered skirt, was an exotic study of perpetual motion as she moved from person to person, chatting about a new play, or discussing her various works- in-progress.

"This is all so exciting, so new to me."

"That's unfortunate," Arina said, her voice suddenly antagonistic again.

Zoe was stunned by the sudden change in her attitude. "I don't understand why you're so angry with me. You act as if everything that's wrong with our world is my fault."

"I don't want to be angry with you, Zoe. But it's difficult to be around your naiveté. The Noncorps are as much a part of the world as the Corporits, or the bloody Aughts, for that matter. We're all here together. This is our planet, too."

"But I've told you before; I've had no involvement with any of this. I couldn't have told you the difference between a Noncorp and a rock."

"I see. Out of sight, out of mind. We might as well not exist as far as most Corporits are concerned." Arina's face flushed an angry red. "And now you're like some damn Corporit out for an afternoon of slumming."

"Arina, stop it, I'm not that way."

"Maybe you're not. But I've spent a good part of my life around Corporits. I know how you people think. I was one of you, remember. Corporits don't care about anyone but themselves. It's an unwritten axiom, a cornerstone of their culture."

"Just because I'm a Corporit doesn't automatically make me your enemy."

"Maybe," Arina said. "But it makes it difficult for us to be friends."

"What about Andrew? And Elliot? You trusted them."

"They were different."

"Maybe I am, too."

Arina nodded thoughtfully. "I hope Andrew's right about you. Since you can't go back, we're sort of stuck with you," she added with a humorless laugh.

* * *

They had been sightseeing for nearly an hour when Zoe's knees buckled. Arina steadied her and steered her to the steps of a nearby building.

"Such a fool," Arina said. "I should have taken you back a long time ago; you're not strong enough yet."

"I want to see more."

"You're not up for this sort of thing."

"I'm all right; the stimulants help," Zoe said, forcing herself to move, to finally stand. "Let's go."

Arina hesitated, but they continued on until the artist stopped in front of a busy shop, where streams of people moved in and out of the entrance.

"Come!" she said, guiding Zoe through the doorway. "Let's take the ambulated walkway."

"Ambulated walkway? Here?"

Arina's belly laughter made Zoe smile.

"Did you think we walked everywhere? We not only have an extensive underground transportation system, we also secretly tap Corporit energy sources to keep it running."

They slid through a revolving door at the back of the shop and into a brick enclosure. Arina centered her second and third fingers on an iridium surface and a metal wall whooshed aside, giving them access to a platform. The door snapped closed behind them with a dull thump.

"Clever!" Zoe said. "It uses the same identification system as Corporit and the CARE units."

"It's a similar DNA activation system," Arina said as they stepped onto a moving belt.

Arina explained that it was part of a vast underground network.

"Corporit leadership knows about our public transportation system, but only unofficially. Consensus is that it would cause more problems than allowing it to continue to operate."

* * *

"End of the line!" the artist said after ten minutes on the beltway. She stepped off, whistling a passage from a Rolfe Z concerto.

"Oh, my God! What is that?"

Zoe stood still and gaped at a huge transparent bubble in their pathway. And there were more of them; bubbles that covered the entire landscape for as far as she could see in every direction. Some were interconnected, others stood as independent hemispheres. But most reached up into the sky and some were at least ten-stories tall.

"These are Asher Wind Storm's Caplac domes."

Zoe was struck by the beauty of the sun shining through the heavy atmosphere, glinting off the domes—a fairyland panorama of iridescent reflections that bounced and dazzled.

"It looks like a massive city of rainbows," she said, turning to Arina. "It is beautiful. But it's much more than that."

"A sea of terrariums?" Zoe said, laughing.

"Very close. But actually, they're vivaria. It's Storm's integrated system to revitalize our earth. The Caplacs contain most of the regional plants and crops that existed before the ecological decimation. Unlike the city domes, here fruit trees grow, blossom, and bear fruit year- round; birds and animals breed and thrive. Every hemisphere is a complete ecosystem. You won't need your nose cannula in there. And these structures are popping up all over the world."

"Like Eden."

Arina smiled at her. “Storm has reenergized extinct flora and produced new species to study how they adapt in the world’s altered environment.”

“How does he do it?”

Arina tugged at her eyes medallion and looked to the sky. “I don’t understand his power, but I do know he’s spent years searching through the last vestiges of the earth’s rain forests, salvaging their genetic secrets. He channels into a universal force that turns barren earth into fertile soil again. The Caplac bubbles provide a safe haven, a place to protect the regenerated life forms from the scorching summer sun, icy winter winds, and destructive pollutants.”

“Like altering basic biochemical reactions.”

“Yes.”

“But with that kind of knowledge, why can’t he do even more, like heal the sick?”

“We can’t heal ourselves if our planet is dying.”

Zoe rubbed hard at her abdomen and glared at Arina. “Sick people, dying people don’t have the luxury of waiting for some perfect time in the future.”

“That’s true,” Arina said. “But when we lost most of the rain forests, our primary source for future curatives was erased. Our world must recover. The past, the present, and the future can’t be separated.” She took Zoe’s arm, walked to the nearest dome.

“I can’t believe the Corporits haven’t stolen this technology from you.”

“Oh, they’ve tried, and they continue to try. But when they cut Storm out of the equation, everything withers and dies.”

“So he won’t work for them?”

“Cooperate, yes. Work for them? Never. Storm rejuvenates the earth for human habitation, not for profit.”

“Clean air? Fresh food? Unpolluted water? Can’t the Corporits share in all of this?”

“Reclamation requires dedicated cooperation. That’s not a concept that suits the Corporit mind.”

"But one person can't heal a planet," Zoe said.

"Storm is a part of a huge network of global Revivers who are creating places like this all over the planet.

"Elliot knew about this?"

"Of course! It's never been a secret. It's simply not something Corporits like to acknowledge. It doesn't fit well into their propaganda machine. It would only bring attention to their own failures. Our dream is to see the domes open to the sky, to see the natural regenerative cycle begin again."

"Like the transportation system."

"Exactly." Arina activated an iridium entry sensor and the doorway snapped open then quickly closed behind them, leaving a seamless skin.

* * *

The aromas hit Zoe first; the wild perfumes of so many plants made her head spin. She reached out and ran her palm across the rough bark of a nearby tree that had grown to the top of the Caplac. She'd only seen trees this size in network video files.

"So this is how the land used to be," Zoe said, scanning the lush landscape in the interior of the gigantic hemisphere. "There were still some forests left when I was very young. But nothing like this." She lifted her nose cannula, breathed in the air and its heavy moisture. It was not only sweet, it seemed alive. She grabbed Arina's hand and hurried forward. She wanted to see more, wanted to feel the warm rays of the sun streaming down between the trees.

The trill of an unseen bird caught her attention; Arina mimicked the call perfectly. The bird dropped to a lower limb. It was almost within reach as it preened its bright yellow feathers and peered curiously at them.

"That's the first bird I've seen outside the zoo since I was a little girl."

"It's pretty amazing, isn't it?"

"How does this man Storm do it? How does he manufacture these structures?" Zoe said as they passed through another dome, and then on to another.

"He relies on the Corporits to produce them to his specifications. Green specifications. The Corporits can accomplish almost anything … except create a stable, democratic social structure."

"Why would they do this for the Noncorps?"

"Your factories will build *anything* for a price."

"But where does Storm get the cash to pay for all of this?"

"He plays the Corporit supply and demand game better than they do." Arina twirled around, opening her arms to the vegetation surrounding them. "Look around you. He has something everyone wants and no one else is able to provide—fresh, naturally grown food."

"He gets them to pay for everything?"

"Everything!."

Zoe looked at the tended fields and orchards. "Who does the labor?"

"I thought you understood—this is a cooperative society. Noncorps, Aughts, and Corporit exiles work side by side. The ecospheres provide shelter and employment for anyone who wants to work."

At the mention of the Aughts, Zoe shivered. "What about the Aughts who attacked Andrew and me?"

"Godan, Tabo, and a few others are isolated savages who don't want to be a part of anything. Storm is their enemy. No matter what we offer, they choose to remain on the outside."

Zoe wandered through forests and glades filled with wildlife, through fields and orchards filled with crops and wildlife she treasured more than anything. Arina followed, gave her the space to explore.

As Zoe watched the mating chase of two squirrels, she lost her balance and stumbled toward an irrigation ditch. A pair of strong hands caught her.

"You wanted to meet Storm again?" Arina said, laughing.

Zoe stared into the familiar amber eyes that had subdued the Aughts.

"It's too soon to be exerting yourself like this," Storm said, looking past Zoe to frown at Arina.

The artist answered him with a shrug and petted the gray wolf that had come to sit beside her.

"I'm so glad you're here. I wanted to see you, to talk with you," Zoe said. "I have so many questions."

Arina waved her on. "Go with Storm. He can show you so much more that I can."

Storm took Zoe's hand as the wolf bounded ahead of them.

* * *

Storm's geodesic home was built with transparent triangles, allowing light to spill in everywhere. The dwelling was deep within the outer protective dome and became a hidden world of its own; a transparent giant mushroom that gave Zoe a 360-degree view of what the world must have been like at one time. She gently touched the leaves of live indoor plants that filled in spaces and accentuated the sparse furnishings. Freestanding bookshelves overflowed with bound volumes.

"I've only read books saved in the electronic networks. I haven't touched an actual book since I was a little girl."

"And most of these are rare and have been deleted from the Corporit network."

She selected a leather bound volume, flipped through the pages, and read aloud, "When I would recreate myself, I seek the darkest wood, the thickest and most interminable, and to the citizen, most dismal swamp. I enter a swamp as a sacred place—a *sanctum sanctorum.* There is the strength, the marrow of Nature."

"Henry David Thoreau," Storm said.

"Who is he?"

"An ancient who loved the earth."

"There's something intimate about holding and reading from a book," she said. "So unlike scanning." Caressing the cover, she lowered herself onto a large pillow.

"Tell me about yourself," he said, pulling up another pillow to sit next to her.

"I'm not very complicated. My life boils down to one simple statement—I can never return to San Francorp."

"That's true."

"Because I have VMAS."

"No, because you'll be eliminated if you return."

"But if Andrew doesn't bring the stabilizer, I'll die here without ever seeing my daughter again."

"There's a place for you here, Zoe. Believe. Envision a different future."

"Why does everyone keep saying that?" she said, tears rolling down her cheeks. "I'm here and my daughter is in San Francorp."

Storm opened his arms and it seemed like the most natural thing to fall into them. She buried her face in his long dark hair and sobbed into his chest.

"Accept the truth."

She pulled away "The truth is, I'm a Corporit. My whole life has been with the Corporits.

My identity is there. My daughter, my world. I don't know anything else." "You can change. There's a place for you here."

"Doing what?"

He dabbed at her tears. "You can treat...you can heal...you can survive." "I'm not sure I can even do that anymore."

"You can."

"And Laya?"

"We'll find a way to get your daughter."

Zoe looked into his eyes, was drawn into their depths. Strange—she barely knew this man, yet she trusted him. And there was something more—her heart was doing a wild dance; leaving her breathless. Before she could think or stop herself, she reached out and touched the leathery skin of his cheek. Her fingers absorbed his memories of harsh cold winters, blistering hot summers.

"I believe you, Storm."

He moved her fingertips to his lips and a wave of warmth washed over her.

Chapter 22

Aught Encampment

Godan swaggered through clots of hunkered men and women. He tasted their bile, smelled their anger, sensed their fear. His spine tingled with suspicion. Their sudden silence when he approached could only mean one thing: they were coming after him; they were going to do him.

He knew the mangy lot, knew their fears; their respect was earned day by day. And losing those Corp'it prisoners to that crazy man had brought not only terror, it had sparked resentment.

And rebellion.

Idiots. All they knew was that Godan hadn't protected them from the man with all those strange powers.

Well, Godan had been in that man's private places. He and others had infiltrated the Eye's bubbles; grabbed food, destroyed underground watering systems; but every time he sneaked into their world, he lost the strongest of his clan—they stayed behind and joined the Eyes. And the Eyes took in the filthy, weak, pieces of shit who wanted the softness and warmth inside the bubbles, who were nothing but dogs who wanted to stay behind instead of return to freedom.

They would leave me so they could work in the dirt with their hands like slaves. Leave me when they could be real men doing as they pleased. Bunch of slugs!

Godan learned to stay away from the bubbles, where the man with the strange eyes stole his men's souls. The clans refused to whisper the man's name, only said he had real,

powerful magic—like wind, earth, fire, or water. Godan laughed at the stupid idiots for believing such shit.

The man they called The Indian was nothing but a trickster.

The dwarf's heart started pounding; his blood raced, throbbed at his temples. He shook with hatred as he studied the faces in the huddled groups around him. He would have to crush the fight in them before they could smother him like the black soot storms that fell from the sky.

Yes, he could beat some of the bastards into submission, even kill a large number of the cowards, but if they were going to remain his, he had to appease them or they would melt away like sludge, maybe even join the clan of his rival, Tabo. Or even worse, would leave to become slaves for the Eyes.

He kicked at different pieces of junk in the piles of garbage and remembered how the Indian and his small group had walked into *his* territory, *his* world, and stole away *his* two prize Corp'it prisoners. And it had been easy for them. What if it had been Tabo, returning to claim more than the two fingers Godan lost the last time they'd fought?

He was roasting from the afternoon heat, but the thought made him shiver.

A whistling hot wind whipped around him and his bones turned to ice; black hatred coursed through his veins when he looked at the others and they stared back at him.

He was alone. No one was on his side.

He thought of his mother. He could still see her steely glower, remember her maniacal resolve. Her face haunted him when he closed his eyes. She had helped him to think, to plan. Why did he kill her? Now he had no one he could trust.

Mean old bitch!

"No-o-o!" he shouted into the wind. "Your fault! Your fault! You shouldn't have taunted me, you ugly hag!" His hands slapped onto his face. Soon he was using a grimy fingernail to pick at a large pimple on the tip of his nose. He squeezed hard at the new eruption and a splat of puss flew into the air.

Agony.

The crush of pain brought a gush of tears and his nose seemed to grow even larger.

Through watery eyes, he watched his people gather scraps of wood for the coming evening fires.

When he studied their lazy movements, he finally understood—the Indian had stolen a special time. He had ripped away their only real entertainment. Now there was nothing but boredom and the same fierce winds, searing days, and bitter cold nights.

And they blamed Godan.

He would have to act now, shift them and their anger away from him. He could take them one at a time, but if they fought together, he was finished.

* * *

Arina Marek left the Caplac dome complex and walked toward the ambulated walkway. Soon she would be back at the Hillsborough Mansionplex.

Departing without saying good-bye to Zoe left her feeling guilty. The woman would learn so much more from Storm. Arina could show her this Noncorp world, but Storm would teach her to survive. He would help her to accept her new life, with its challenges, in a way Arina never could.

It was difficult to let go when she was still was at odds with herself about the female doctor. Could she really trust this woman?

Trusting any Corporit was extremely difficult for Arina. But she acknowledged her deep- seated bias and would never turn away anyone seeking refuge, especially those who had escaped from Corporit's Desisto Program.

Zoe had been one of those people marked for death.

She remembered Elliot Hidalga. He had been a valuable member of the Defys, subverting the Corporit medical system at every opportunity. He'd saved many, many lives and Arina wanted to believe that he would have only chosen the best as a companion. And Andrew's friendship with the woman was an important factor to consider.

Could she simply be jealous of Zoe?

Jealous of what? The fact she was younger? More beautiful?

No. The woman was sick with VMAS. Her body was wasted, her arms a crazy quilt of ugly purple blotches.

Envy?

Her memory picked at the vision of Storm carrying Zoe into her Hillsborough home, cradling her as he would one of his wounded animals. She'd seen the passion in his eyes, and it was there again when they met today.

That wasn't Storm the mystic, the Earth healer, the reviver. That was Storm the man, the human, the lover.

And he desired Zoe.

Didn't he protect me, take me under his wing, love me after I fled the Corporits all those years ago? Didn't he save me when I was on the brink of self-destruction?

Today, they enjoyed a different kind of love. But she missed his closeness and suffered the pangs of regret in remembering how both their passions had cooled to become a bonding friendship.

Two Aughts suddenly stood in her way as she approached the entrance to the ambulated walkway. She'd been too lost in her thoughts to catch a whispered command, a scurry of feet.

Recognizing Godan, she turned and ran back toward the domes. Another pair of Aughts blocked the path.

"Where's the Corp'its that asshole and his followers stole from me?" Godan shouted, pointing toward the domes with the handle of a coiled whip.

"You're out of your garbage pit, little man," Arina said, looking down at the dwarf, who was half her size. She planted her feet and jammed her fists tightly against her hips.

The men turned and looked at Godan. A couple of them snickered. "Too big for you?"

Godan silenced them with a glare. He stepped toward Arina, lashing out with the whip; it coiled, like a snake, around her neck. He yanked at it until she was down on her knees, coughing and choking.

Arina scrambled in the dirt, her eyes always on Godan. As he moved hand-over-hand along the length of the whip, she struggled to remain steady on her knees. When their faces were within a few inches of each other, she spat in his eyes.

"You whore!" he shouted, grabbing a fistful of her hair to

wipe the spit away. Then he yanked the noose tighter.

"This one will do," he yelled. "One uppity bitch is as good as another."

* * *

The four Aughts beat and kicked the woman during the long trek back to Godan's territory. The campfires were lit and the Aughts began to gather. The crowd stared in stony silence at Godan and his new prize.

The whip was still laced around the large woman's neck, but she held her head high, and returned the curious looks of the crowd, even smiled at the smaller children.

Godan stomped back and forth, uncomfortable with the silence. Had he been wrong? Had he misjudged them?

"What's with all of you?" he screamed, shaking a fist. "The Indian stole what was ours with six men. Today we evened the score, with only four of us at risk. Isn't this what you wanted?"

Heads began to nod.

Godan drew his knife, slashed away at Arina's clothes. Within seconds, she stood naked before them. Rivulets of blood trailed across her skin.

"Look at the tits on her," yelled a toothless man.

"She's got enough ass for two of us," screamed another.

The catcalls became a chant. Children giggled and darted forward to pinch Arina's legs and kick at her feet. Godan leered, raked his pointed nails across her breasts, leaving behind more weeping beads of blood. He yanked on the whip, bringing her head down to him.

"Call me a little man, will you," he shouted into her ear.

When she straightened, he smeared the trails of blood up and down and across her body.

The crowd became a single roar.

Arina looked at the mottled sky, then glanced down at Godan.

"You *are* a little man; smaller than the smallest pimple in that festering nest on your mangy nose."

The Aughts roared with laughter.

Drool ran down Godan's chin, hatred crushed his eyes to slits as he beat her with his fists.

The roar from the crowd was like a frenzy of fiery sparks shooting into the sky.

"Godan! Godan! Godan!"

The dwarf smiled at his subjects, spat at Arina.

"Kill the bitch! Take her fingers! Kill the bitch!"

Arina disconnected from the pain that screamed from every part of her body. She soared above the seething masses, envisioned Storm's promised journey. She climbed higher and higher, spinning away from the last of the earthbound cries.

"Killthebitch-killthebitch-killthebitch!"

Godan danced around and around Arina, shaking a winner's fist over his head. The crowd roared as he sliced off the index and middle finger of each hand, raised his knife high in the air, and plunged it into her heart again and again.

Chapter 23

The Domes

First Andrew, then Arina, and now Storm. Each had said the same thing:

You can't go back!

Their words continued to echo in Zoe's head.

You can't go back. You can't go back.

Until now, she'd refused to accept the basic reality of that simple statement. But how long could she hide from the truth?

Corporit identity? It had been her beginnings. Her roots. Her life. Everything she'd ever known since she was very young had its origins with the Corporits. She'd accepted and lived by their code. She may have questioned many of their precepts, but she'd never thought of herself as a rebel; she still found it difficult to believe that soft spoken Elliot had been a Defy.

Her mother had been a believer in the Corporit system—she taught Corporit political science at the university. Zoe remembered many arguments between her mother and father at the dinner table. He was a soil engineer and ranted about the damage to the basic structure of the planet and the destruction of its ecosystem. Zoe remembered leaving the table when their arguments became so intense they would scream at each other. Then they wouldn't speak to each other for days. Zoe would try to ignore both of them and dream about being a physician someday…someone who could help other people.

That dream didn't come true, at least not in any way I can relate to.

Storm's world?

Community, people helping each other. Revival of our planet.

Maybe she could be a Reviver, someone who actively cherished the earth. Could this be a world of beginnings? A world of hope?

Maybe she could be healthy and strong again in this world. Maybe this *was* a good place to bring Laya, not just as a place to hide, but a place to really live. Maybe they could turn their backs on the Corporit world and its restricted way of life.

Maybe.

Storm had left her to explore the domes. He must have known she needed time to absorb the possibilities open to her. She pressed her fingers to an iridian doorplate and stepped into a massive citrus orchard, inhaled the heady scents of orange blossoms. The perfume in the air kept breaking into her thoughts. She picked a flower from the nearest cluster and stuck it behind her ear.

Asher Wind Storm!

Had she ever known a man like him? He'd not only saved her life, he'd become an anchor. Someone real, someone solid to hang onto.

She wandered from dome to dome, marveling at everything she saw, from the smallest creature to the largest tree.

Now, she was in a rolling vineyard that stretched as far as she could see. The closest vines were heavy with mature fruit. She snapped off a small bunch of grapes and held them up to the light. The purple iridescence contrasted sharply with the ugly blotches on her arm.

Had they faded?

At first, she thought it was the diminishing light, but as she looked closer, she saw the telltale coloration *had* changed.

Remission?

Don't be a fool, Zoe Hidalga!

There was no recorded evidence of spontaneous VMAS remission.

Stop the fantasies. They won't change a thing.

If there was any hope for her—real hope—it was getting the stabilizing compound. If it didn't work? Perhaps the Corporit policy of quickly ending her life was the better solution.

She moved into a pine forest. Like the orange orchard, the

aromas were intoxicating.

How safe, how insulated she was at this moment. If there were any answers, they might be here, where birds darted back and forth as the sun dropped lower in the sky.

The sudden movement of the gray wolf that emerged from the forest startled her. She knew she had found her way back to Storm's dome. The wolf stood staring at her.

Soft music echoed through the woods. Reedy vibrations made her breath catch. The wolf came to her, allowed itself to be petted, then turned and wandered down the path, looking back at her. She followed it to a small glade and saw Storm silhouetted by the setting sun. Even through the thick atmosphere, it seemed as though the sky was shooting flames.

She could barely breathe as she listened to the intensity of the music coming from the small set of panpipes that he held delicately in both hands. The wolf loped ahead and settled down beside him.

She stood knee deep in a patch of tall, wild grass to listen to notes that were like arrows that pierced her heart with their beauty. He turned to her, amber eyes soft, yet, at the same time, intense. An unexpected thrill clutched her groin. His music swelled in a crescendo, then descended to the softest of trills before rising again.

Storm's soft brown hair clung to his neck. He bent his head in concentration. Zoe's eyes swept across his strong arms; his skin seemed to glow. She couldn't help swaying to the unfamiliar rhythm as he stood and moved toward her. His eyes searched hers, eyes that reflected compassion and love, eyes filled with something else, something she was afraid to understand. When he stood beside her, the notes quickened, became urgent, lifted her high above the forest, the vineyards, the orchards; then carried her even higher…and higher.

She felt so alive. Whole. Free!

The sounds suddenly dropped into a grating growl. The wolf stood protectively in front of Zoe and Storm and the flaming sky fragmented into a sea of flickering lights that washed through the woods.

Zoe tensed at the sight of approaching Noncorp torchbearers. In their midst, a cart held a limp body.

"No!" Storm cried.

Zoe's heart pounded hard. She recognized the long flowing hair with purple accents. She cried out, "Arina!"

They lifted the body from the cart and laid it down among a grove of seedling redwoods. Some of them began to dig a grave in the fertile soil; others tenderly cleansed away all traces of the blood and dirt that smeared across her nakedness. The battered and lacerated body told a terrible story of her last moments. Every part of her body had been violated. Zoe knew the significance of the missing second and third fingers from each hand. Godan's name was carved deep into the flesh of one arm.

Storm sat at the head of the open grave; the wolf keened next to him. They wrapped the artist in layers of multicolored shawls and gently lowered her into the ground. Everyone turned to Storm.

"Today, our sister returns to the universe from which we all sprang," Storm said.

The crowd nodded its agreement.

"Her mortal remains will nourish this fledgling grove of redwoods, which she loved with all her heart. They will grow so they can tower over all living things as their ancestors did many decades ago. And as they grow taller and stronger, they will remind us that Arina Marek was a rare giant among us."

Everyone sobbed. Zoe shared not only their tears, but their anger. Godan's clan was a harsh symptom of how the Corporits had spread hatred like a noxious disease. It affected every form of life. Zoe silently vowed to become the kind of person Arina would have been proud to call her friend.

Storm lifted the pipes to his lips. The air carried a mournful harmonic tune skyward as the sun dipped below the horizon.

* * *

In the darkening sky, a huge cloud formed, swirled in all directions—north, south, east, and west. Eventually, it hovered restlessly over a massive bonfire where a triumphant Godan and his drunken followers danced around roaring flames.

The black cloud morphed into twin amber eyes that filled with tears at the sight of the celebration.

One of the Aughts, struck by a falling drop of water, looked up, shouted, and pointed at the sky. Others staggered in confusion as a cascade of salty tears fell. Rivulets formed in the dry earth, rapidly swelling into rushing streams that snuffed out Godan's victory bonfire.

The deluge was relentless. It inundated the Aughts, seared wounds, opened sores. Shouted obscenities only intensified the pain.

Godan watched Arina Marek's severed fingers dissolve at his feet; all traces flowed away in a rush. He shrieked skyward.

"I did it, you fucking earth-digger! And I'll do you, too, if I get the chance!"

A jagged spear of white-hot lightning slashed across the sky and struck into the midst of the huddled, half-drowned Aughts. They were flung in all directions, screaming as they clawed at their burning chests, all now etched with the words:

ARINA LIVES.

Chapter 24

Noncorp Sector

Zoe and Storm sat high upon a hill that separated two distinct worlds. Looking toward San Francorp, Zoe saw the Corporit spread of land. It was nothing but a massive void with the constant swirl of wind-borne dust. Zoe followed the sweep of Storm's hand as he took in the Corporit emptiness.

"If Earth's inhabitants follow their present destructive path," Storm said, "our world will become an empty rock, a lifeless planet that will wander in a predetermined orbit through the vast universe. Lifeless. Silent."

In the opposite direction, she watched a new Caplac environment being created. The empty shell waited for the birth of a new world.

On the inside of the dome, Storm explained, workers were treating the soil with heavy compost. They could see that the Caplac inner skin was soaked with moisture exuding from the hot primal mixture.

Zoe and Storm became silent. She knew the sound of their voices could destroy not only a precious moment of contemplation, but also a journey into a spiritual place she had little knowledge of. But it was Storm's world; a place she wanted to enter and comprehend.

Storm said, "I come here to study, to try to understand the mysteries of life, to see the beginning and the end in one breath." He looked toward the horizon. "Arina and I came here together many times."

"I wanted to know her better," Zoe said. "I never realized our time would be so brief."

"Time is eternal, yet it remains our worst enemy. " Storm looked into her eyes. "Arina knew that better than most."

"Tell me about her."

Storm fingered away a wisp of Zoe's hair from her eyes,

wrapped an arm around her, and held her close to him.

"When Arina came to live with us, she was a bitter, burned-out nurse running away from Corporit medicine. They'd just started the depopulation program and she wanted no part of it."

"She said she'd never been an artist until she came here."

Storm smiled. "People were drawn to her. I was drawn to her."

"The two of you were lovers?"

"Long, long ago. But right from the start, she was my friend. That never changed."

"In just the brief time I've been here, I've begun to feel a sense of hope. Arina was helping me to understand so many things—that maybe I *can* raise my daughter, that I *can* hope for a tomorrow. Arina tried to tell me that, wanted me to believe it."

"She was a wise woman." His attention, his voice drifted away for a moment. Then he whispered, "We came together to heal our loneliness."

"But people love you," she said. "There isn't a person here who wouldn't die for you."

"No one has to die for me. Time will take care of that."

"You seem so powerful, beyond loneliness, beyond even death."

Storm laughed. The sound circled the air around them. "No one is beyond the empty spaces within or the blackness beyond. The cycle of life and its journey always has a beginning and an end. It's a part of the great mystery."

"And your journey?" Zoe said. "How did it begin?"

Storm ran his fingers through the sterile dirt as though he was willing it to life.

"My mother was a scientist…a chemist. She raised me by herself, wouldn't tell me anything about my father other than to say he was a full-blooded Maricopa, and that he was dead."

"What happened to her, to your mother?"

Storm smiled at her. "My mother filled me with awe and a curiosity about life. Yet, she was one of the first Desisto casualties. She had the power to heal herself, but she always counseled that her power would fade as mine grew." Storm looked away. "And she was right…but that was a very long time ago."

"Where were you when she died?"

"I was away at a Corporit university. She never once told me her heart was failing, but I should have known something was wrong. I could have helped her." Storm covered his eyes. "Every dome I build I dedicate to her. She taught me that the universe is a powerful place…that it has secrets, some of which she revealed to me. She showed me that all secrets can be tapped into, that I must continue to search, to find the answers to save our dying world."

Zoe laid her head down on his shoulder. She felt at peace, safe.

Soon their fingers entwined, and then they kissed.

Chapter 25

Robotic OR – Theater One

Andrew Potter stood outside the decontamination area; he was the last of four surgeons to enter for a pre-surgical scrub down. It was all he could do not to turn tail and run.

When the light over the doorway flashed green, he stepped through the entry, stripped, and neatly hung his clothes in a sealed closet.

He briefly examined the wound on his shoulder.

It was an angry red and the sutures had loosened enough to guarantee he would end up with a wide, ugly scar. But the thigh laceration was by far the worst of the two. It went clear to the bone, forcing him to take long-term massive antibiotics to prevent problems that he didn't dare think about.

He cringed as he walked into the chamber and heard the loud hiss that secured him inside; the room was now tight as a tomb. A series of deep breaths helped him take in the rich flow of oxygen that blew on his face. Normally it would have given him a momentary lift, but at the same time, a stinging solution sprayed every inch of his body.

Both of his wounds started screaming in unison when the scrubbers began their methodical rub over his body. He tried to escape the equipment by moving to the farthest corner of the chamber, not only to avoid the scrubbing, but also the air pressure jets that pounded and probed his cuts and wounds, along with the rest of his body. But the highly sensitive sterilization equipment was geared to his personal body temperature and followed him with the tenacity of a predator determined to skin him alive.

He thought of his ex-wife and how she would have used his torn muscles as an example of how he risked his life, not only for friendship, but for a cause that could end his relentless scientific search for answers to physical regeneration through cybernetics.

Because she'd asked, he'd almost given up his Defy involvement. And right now, when every part of his body was in pain, he wondered if she'd been right. Maybe this dangerous political endeavor *was* asking too much of him.

He could still see her face; soft skin, violet eyes, generous lips that smiled in that special way. Why couldn't she have believed that truly the most passionate involvement in his life was still always going to be her? A sharp pain that had nothing to do with his injuries slashed through him. She'd been gone for a year now and he'd heard she was in a new relationship. Unexpected tears sprang from his eyes. He still missed her every single day.

After the required ten-minute skin sterilization, a door opened and he was admitted to the surgical area. The room was small, dedicated to injuries and special procedures that required few working personnel. The walls were that strange pewter color composed of polymers with tight molecular configurations to discourage bacterial or viral penetration. There was a single patient table with two trays to hold necessary instruments.

It was the safest place in the building for Defy cell meetings and updates. Each rebel cell was limited to four people, and they all had to work in the same corporation so that any gathering would appear normal or expected.

Of course, the pre-op procedure forced all of them to undergo the unnecessary ten-minute body scrub, and it was a lot to ask since they hadn't come there to perform surgery. But no one complained. Some things were more important than inconvenience, even discomfort or pain from air brushes roughing you. Besides, with this method, the chances of any listening device being present or brought in by a mole was virtually nil—going through decontamination would destroy any communicator or listening device. Even their ears were washed and scrubbed with special filaments and solutions.

The Defy protective structure and management was based on survival logic. And logic was something Andrew not only understood, but had complete faith in.

Although they were now in a secure environment, the Defy members of this cell never referred to each other by name. Each of them was designated A, B, C, or D just in case some kind of listening device did make its way into the meeting. Andrew was A.

He could see that every one of the three waiting, naked surgeons made a point of evaluating his body wounds. All of them mirrored surprise and alarm that dug new lines of concern in their faces.

D was the first to comment. “What happened, A?”

C piped in, “Those are serious injuries. Who did that to you?”

B remained silent, waiting for Andrew to answer the two previous questions.

Andrew saw each one of them was genuinely worried about his physical condition; he couldn’t just dismiss it or refuse to answer. Besides, he knew they wouldn’t let it go without an explanation.

“Look, I was helping a friend escape to the Noncorp area,” he finally said. “She’s been DP listed, and if I didn’t help her, she’d have been caught and sanctioned.”

D was angry. “You have no business getting involved with that kind of personal business.

It’s too dangerous. Your obligation is to Defy.”

“She’s an old friend, the wife of Elliot Hidalga. You remember him, don’t you?”

“I certainly do remember him, C said. “He was a tireless organizer when we were first coming together.” He thought for a moment, then added, “He died of VMAS, didn’t he?”

“Yes. And now Zoe has it also.”

“Why wasn’t she DP sanctioned immediately?” D was infuriated.

“She went to a CARE unit for diagnosis and then she called me.”

B looked at Andrew, his eyes wide. “A CARE unit? Then the CAPOs are after her—”

D interrupted. "There's not much you can do for her now anyway. She'll be dead soon. It wasn't worth the risk."

"Zoe's my friend. I could never turn her away."

"Those wounds," D said, pointing first at Andrew's shoulder, then at his thigh. "How exactly did you get them?"

"We were captured by the Aughts."

"Jeez, you're going to need every antibacterial and antiviral aid we can throw at you," C said. "Those people are nothing but disease buckets. How the hell did you get away from those animals?"

"Asher Wind Storm."

They were suddenly excited. B jumped in. "How? What did he do?"

"I don't really know. I passed out and when I woke up, I was in the central Noncorp area."

They started peppering him with questions. When he refused to answer anymore, they finally relaxed and smiled at each other as they stood around without a stitch of clothing on their bodies. They were all long past lewd remarks about body imperfections, having long ago accepted this was the only way to get into the OR safely for the necessary exchange of information. Sticking to established routine protocols were essential; turning off or avoiding he decontamination process would leave an anomaly in the system. Someone would be required to look into it, evaluate it, and generate a report.

All of them worked in the Robotic Division so no one would question their motives for being in an OR. Surgeons were expected to meet, to process, integrate, and demonstrate their individual techniques. It was a necessary part of their professional goals and education.

B said, "Let's get on with it."

C said, "I'm happy to report that Defy infiltration and sabotage is now at its highest peak in five years."

"And so is our membership," B said. "It's really exciting."

"It's as if everyone has been asleep for thirty years since the Corporit takeover," D said. "And they're now waking up and taking a hard look at our society and the disintegrating world the Corporits created."

"And they don't like what they see," Andrew said. "I've heard people ask how they can join our movement in open conversations. Somehow, we're going to have to make ourselves more accessible. We need everyone on our side."

D shook his head. "And some of those people wanting in could be Corporit spies. I still think we have to keep the leaders under cover. If the Corporits can pinpoint our leadership, they can make a concerted effort to wipe us out."

"You're right, D. But it's still exciting. We've worked so hard to change this rotten system," C said.

"Within a year, we'll have moles planted in all the news and propaganda corporations," Andrew said. "That's absolutely essential. It's the only way to reach all the people."

"And when the Corporit National Council is finally crushed," D said. "All communications will be in Defy hands during the transition."

"We'll have to put CNC down. Without them, it will make taking control and tossing the Corporits out a lot easier," added B.

"Hopefully, with communications open again, more and more people will join us from every part of the world," Andrew said. "Our rebellion has to survive."

Andrew moved to the operating table, the others followed. They encircled the anatomically complete Surgiclone. Today's procedure would have demonstrated delicate brain stem surgery. Although it was very tricky operation, only one neurosurgeon and a highly sophisticated robot would be necessary to perform the tricky task. Andrew opened the instrument pack and handled the array of specialized tools. If someone decided to check up on them, the pack will look like it had been used for the demonstration. There should be no trail of complications or questions about their meeting.

That's the way Andrew liked it.

Zoe and her problems couldn't have happened at a worse

time. There's very little I can personally do for her now. Can't risk everything the Defys have worked so hard to achieve.

He nodded at everyone and they closed the meeting.

* * *

The file of Dr. Andrew Potter, chief of Robotics, filled Dutton's screen. A scan of the doctor's current profile and activities had been anonymously posted by one of his deepest-undercover agents. There was no note, only the file.

Dutton scrolled down:

FRIEND: ELLIOT HIDALGA
DEFY SUSPECT—VMAS—DELAYED DP—
HOME TREATMENT.
NOTE: POTTER INTERROGATION RE
HIDALGA—NEGATIVE SUBVERSIVE
ACTIVITIES OR CONNECTIONS
UNCOVERED

An automatic alert filled the screen.

ZOE HIDALGA—WIFE OF ELLIOT HIDALGA—
VMAS—DP—AT LARGE

Well, what have we here, Dr. Potter?

Hmmm, Potek's secret arrangement for undercover work is finally paying off.

Dutton scanned the doctor's complete biography, skimming through most of the lengthy history that began with Potter as a child genius…brilliant student…innovative mind. Noncorp CARE units originated from Potter's paradigm—a framework for independent robotic diagnosis and treatment. Dutton could see that the man probably had few rivals in creating robotic brain surgery.

One of a kind, eh?

Dutton hated geniuses. They always seemed so indispensable. But he knew better. He could get rid of every one of them, and there would always be another can't-do-without-wonder to fill the slot.

On the surface, the doctor appeared to be a genuine Corporit star, a rare person who totally submerged all his energies into his work. It was the only real passion that Dutton uncovered about Potter as he plundered the history banks of the computer files.

And buying his time from Robotics had been a good investment for Medi-Prog. Too bad any replacement would cost Dutton's corporation large sums of extra money. The board wouldn't be tolerant of anything that hurt profits.

I need to prove, without a doubt, that Potter is a traitor.

Reading the file suggested there definitely was something about Potter that raised a pink, if not red, flag. The Hidalga connection seemed to be the greatest weakness at present. Was Potter helping Zoe Hidalga, the missing DP?

Maybe it's time for everyone to stop being blinded by Potter's genius and put some real surveillance on our genius friend, see if it produces anything to explain why I received a computer alert that Potter may have strayed from the straight and narrow. Is our revered robotics doctor guilty of something more serious than iffy relationships?

He picked up his private communicator and punched in a familiar and often used number.

* * *

George Potek stood at attention in front of Dutton's desk. His eyes were fixed straight ahead, purposely avoiding looking directly at Dutton. Potek always seemed to know when Dutton was in one of his no-nonsense moods.

"Potek, sit down!"

"Yes sir!" He slid into the chair opposite Dutton, but he still looked rigid, like he had a rod up his ass.

"What do you have on Andrew Potter?"

"The chief of Robotics?" Potek said, looking surprised.

"Aren't you the brilliant one?" Dutton said, "Yes, the chief of Robotics."

"Just routine surveillance, but nothing special," Potek said. "At this time he isn't a person of interest."

"Your undercover person says there may be reason to change that status. I want a constant eye on him, and I want him brought in for Stage One questioning." Dutton slid to the edge of his chair, stood, and began to pace around his office.

Potek removed a notebook and pen from an inside jacket pocket, watched attentively. "Still using paper, I see," Dutton said. "What's wrong with a Doculslate?"

Potek mumbled, "Just used to this, sir."

Dutton continued to pace.

He was irritated even though he had no real reason or solid evidence for looking into Potter other than a vague connection to a dead friend and the man's wife, who was now a DP on the loose. And he knew Potter was too well known for him to get away with a formal interrogation at this point.

"Is there anything specific you're suspicious about?" Potek said.

Dutton stopped mid-stride. "Do I have to explain *everything* to you, Potek? Just do what I tell you."

Potek was silent, but nodded.

"Who's the one with the brains here? Who's the one in charge?"

"You are, sir." Potek's voice had lost some of its timbre. "But it helps if we can have some sense of what you might be looking for…what your suspicions might be."

"So now I'm supposed to do your job for you?"

"No, sir I only meant—"

"Dammit, stop sputtering."

"Yes sir."

Dutton slipped back into his seat, picked up a pen, and began tapping it against the desktop.

"Will that be all, sir?"

"I'll decide when this meeting is over, you idiot." Dutton's voice had dropped to a level of menace that made even *him* take notice.

It was obvious George Potek was cowed. He stared at Dutton with a shamed expression, but Dutton felt uneasy about his demeanor. Potek was one of the few people he could confide in, could trust without reservation, and he'd just acted like an ass to him.

"Oh, relax, Potek. I'm just having a bad day. It has nothing to do with you." Potek's response was to sit up taller in his seat, the rod in place again.

"I can't put my finger on it, but something is not quite right about our brilliant Dr. Potter.

Maybe he's too perfect. Too much of a star."

"We'll check him out, sir."

"Yes, you do that. As soon as possible.

* * *

Nathan Quinn sat at his desk, his concentration shot. No matter how hard he tried to go about his work, his mind kept drifting into melodic reveries. He hummed long forgotten songs, notes he hadn't sung in years. Poems floated through his head and he could actually visualize the words printed on a page in a book he hadn't looked at since he was a teenager.

Had he been on a drinking binge?

No, he'd only had one glass of wine with Seka. At least that's all he could remember.

He mentally backtracked—the earlier part of yesterday was clear, every detail of it. There were the various meetings he'd attended; there was Emory Dutton's pointed interest and obvious suspicion of him; there was the anticipation, the excitement of seeing Seka, selecting the wine, finding the scarce repli-roses.

It was strange though, that he couldn't remember anything after he'd arrived at Seka's apartment. Maybe he *did* have more than one drink. And if so, why didn't he remember?

Whatever had actually happened during those hours was now lost, hidden behind a gauzy curtain that opened and closed at random, but never all the way.

"Damn!" After three attempts, he still couldn't bring up a run-of-the-mill report on the computer. His sluggish fingers refused to go where he wanted them to go. And he was sweltering, burning up with stabbing spikes of heat. Worst of all, he kept fighting a crazy compulsion to repeat his own name over and over as though he might become disoriented and forget who he was.

This is insane.

A flash of memory superimposed itself on the monitor: Seka, her body open, moist, smooth legs wrapped around him. She was so beautiful.

He couldn't believe he'd been fired by passion strictly tied to physical attraction. It wasn't like him. He'd always wanted more than just sex. The women he slept with were usually intellectually challenging and although Seka *was* intelligent; he couldn't recall one word of their conversation. But he had a vivid recollection of her breasts, her curves, the feel of her, the taste of her; how she moved beneath him.

But not one word of what they'd said to one another.

His body betrayed his noble thoughts about intellectual stimulation as he responded to another fleeting image of the night's bedroom gymnastics. He looked around to see if anyone was watching. Had he ever shared such erotic surrender, such uninhibited passion?

He breathed deeply, tried to shrug off his pounding headache, and stared at the computer screen again. His fingers moved to the keys. A string of alerts flashed into sight.

Scanning the scrolled information, he jammed a finger onto the freeze key and stared at the monitor:

ZOE HIDALGA
STAT PHARMCORP ORDER

How can there be a purchase order for a DP?

But then, there was the basic Corporit law regarding commerce:

No entity may interfere with the sale of product.
Free trade is the foundation of Corporit existence.

The entry time for the order was close to two hours ago. He scrolled back to find the generated order:

CODE 003135 X66
RECOMB II.

He quickly brought up the Personnel Code Index, which told him that Code 003135 was Andrew Potter, MD, Director of Robotic Medicine.

Who is this guy and what's he up to!

Nathan keyed a query to Pharmcorp to find out the classification and action/kinetics of X66.

CLASSIFIED: NTKO

Need to know only?

He tried again.

CLASSIFIED: NTKO

Only someone like Emory Dutton could directly enter that kind of file. He tried a different tactic and called up the Desisto Status Report. He held his breath as he keyed in Zoe's name.

ZOE HIDALGA: DESISTO PROCESS STATUS—AT LARGE.

My God. She must still be alive. Where the devil is she?

"Damn!"

He spun around in his chair, saw Seka standing in the doorway. He hadn't meant to comment out loud.

"Problems?" she asked, looking past him to see what was on his monitor.

Nathan reached back and deleted the information. He didn't dare take a chance of her or anyone else seeing this.

"Just the usual boring review of AM reports."

"Oh? Do you always talk to the computer?" she said, laughing.

"And other inanimate objects on occasion." His words were lighthearted but he couldn't take his eyes off of her.

"Hope you enjoyed the evening as much as I did," she said.

"It made coming back to work this morning difficult, if not almost impossible."

"M-m-m. I know what you mean."

He tapped the desktop with his fingertips. "And speaking of work, could you have someone get us a printout on CARE unit accuracy for the past twelve months?

"When do you need it?"

"Before noon, if possible. And I'd appreciate it if you would check it first for any anomalies."

"What are you looking for?"

"I'm not really sure. Just a hunch there's a glitch somewhere in the system."

When Seka returned to her unit, Nathan left his office, started for the lounge, looking into each of the cramped cubicles along the way. Medi-Prog positions had a high level of turnover. It wouldn't be difficult to find a vacant office from which to make his call.

He looked around. No one seemed to being paying attention to him.

At the first empty slot, he slipped inside and dialed Andrew Potter's number on the inter- office telelink. The line was busy.

"Come on! Come on!"

He pressed the repeat signal button over and over until the telelink connected.

"Yeah?" a gruff voice responded at the other end.

Nathan could hear angry shouts in the background.

"Is this Dr. Andrew Potter's office?" he asked.

"Identify yourself!"

Nathan disconnected and immediately left the cubicle.

Chapter 26

Cable Car Conglomerate
Dr. Andrew Potter's Apartment

CAPO Commander George Potek was on the spot again with the volatile Medi-Prog CEO. The man treated him like an idiot, invaded his life night and day, and kept Potek constantly on edge. He chewed on a thumbnail, clutched the telelink, and listened.

Emory Dutton's voice echoed harshly through the earpiece. "Well, anything yet, Commander?"

"No, sir. As you know, we've already checked his office and it appears there's nothing here in his apartment, either. I think Potter's in the clear."

"Think? Did I ask you to think?"

Potek jerked the communicator away from his ear, held it at arm's length as the CEO screamed at him. "*I* think Potter's up to something. That's why I've had him picked up, you idiot. That's why he's here in interrogation."

"Yes, sir." Potek tried to grab a deep breath, shoved a finger between his collar and neck.

"Bring me some evidence so I can put this traitor away." Dutton's voice had finally come down a few decibels. "I can't legally hold the bastard here much longer."

"Sir, I have my best team on it. If he's into something, we'll find it."

But the line was dead. Dutton had already hung up.

Potek's stomach clenched until he thought he would retch. This was why there was no woman in his life, why he had so few friends. This was why he lived alone, with work as his only companion. Each and every time he thought he'd found someone to share his life, she turned around and left. Every one of the women complained to Potek, said the CAPOs were his life. There was no room in his world for anyone else.

And they were right. And so was Dutton.

Think? He didn't need to think. He just needed to do his job so his corporation remained at the top of the list for this sector's security. Keep up the stats that showed no other corporation was even a close second. Potek might yearn for the time to find love or friendship, but the reality was that he would always have to give the CAPOs his constant attention, his everything, if the corporation was to remain number one.

Potek turned to watch his squad continue their search through Potter's living accommodations.

"These hot shots live in luxury while the rest of us are forced into cells," muttered Corporal Adam Lutz. Clothes scattered everywhere when he up-ended a drawer and let it crash to the floor.

"Something bothering you, Corporal Lutz?" Potek shouted, glaring at the man.

"No, sir!" Lutz snapped to attention.

"Get on with it then. No one gives a rat fuck about your running commentary on Dr. Potter's lifestyle."

"Yes, Commander."

"Anyone else have anything to say?" Silence.

Potek knew his staff, could spot a troublemaker by sniffing the air. Lutz had a big mouth.

He could cause Potek problems. Better to deal with it now.

"All right. Get it out in the open!" Potek shouted. Six heads turned to Lutz as the Commander waited for a response.

The corporal spoke up. "We've been promised larger living quarters for more than a year, sir. The wife keeps nagging at me day and night about being squeezed into one room. This guy ..." his hand waved back and forth ..."lives like a king. One single person with a living room and two bedrooms. And that meter-less shower. Shit, I'd give my left nut for it."

Potek sneered. "You're a grunt, Lutz. Andrew Potter is chief of Robotic Surgery. Makes sense, doesn't it?"

"Not really," Niya Axton said, removing her dark glasses.

Potek looked at the woman. Her captives always came in battered, sometimes bloodied.

She liked to push perps around. But to her credit, no one ever escaped on her watch.

"We put our lives on the line every single day," Axton continued. "Isn't that worth something?"

"Yeah, three meals and a roof over your head. But I wouldn't want any of you doing surgery on me," Potek said with a straight face. "You're good, but not that good."

The four other members of the group kept silent, their eyes skipping back and forth between the speakers, like watching a ping-pong match.

"We live in a corporacracy, and don't you forget it. Each of you can be replaced with another grunt in the blink of an eye. And if you don't like your job or the way things are done, hoof it out to the Noncorp area."

"Is that what you really want?" Lutz blurted.

"Doesn't matter what I want." Potek picked up the battered drawer and handed it back to Lutz. "Fact is, I've got plenty of others ready to take your place…in a heartbeat."

"Still seems unfair," Axton said.

"Go ahead. Transfer out if you want." Potek laughed at their grim faces. "Maybe you can even snatch up a better gig, like cleaning out city sewers. And there's always toxic waste transport. They're always on the lookout for people."

"Sir!" Axton said.

Potek ignored her. "How about the nuclear fuel disposal dumps?" He pulled at his earlobe, smiled. "Those guys? They have a life expectancy of two years. Tops!"

Lutz and Axton exchanged glances. "No, sir. That won't be necessary," Lutz said.

"Good. How about you, Axton?"

"Our CAPO unit is just fine with me, sir."

"I thought so." Potek moved to the window, looked down at the street. "Now get your asses back to work and see if we can find at least *something* suspicious about this fat cat."

Chapter 27

CAPO Headquarters
Interrogation Unit

The look of terror on Andrew's assistant's face when Andrew entered the department's outer reception area warned him that something was wrong, very wrong.

He walked inside his office, where three CAPOs awaited him. Pictures of his mother and father were tossed aside and the single picture he kept of his ex-wife, usually hidden inside a drawer, was now on top of his desk among a jumble of computer printouts from several notebooks containing early robotic schematics. The CAPOs apparently had gone through every drawer and shelf in his office. And they seemed to have made a point of not being neat about it.

Even though there was nothing incriminating to be found, a rush of fear made Andrew's heart crash against his chest. He could barely breathe.

"You're coming with us, Doctor," the head CAPO said. One of his men yanked Andrew's arm, sending a spike pain to his injured shoulder.

"What's this about? What's the charge?"

Without a word, they rushed him out of the building, stuffed him into a vehicle, and hauled him to CAPO headquarters, where he was shoved into a mirrored room with nothing but a high plastin stool in the center. He sat down, but with no lower footrest, the weight of his dangling leg pulled hard at his sutures, threatening to rip open his thigh wound. He was weak and bone weary. He wanted to stand, to move around, but he was afraid he'd fall flat on his face.

This whole thing had to be about Zoe Hidalga. He knew they might come for him. Ordering the restricted VMAS stabilizing compound for her was a huge risk. After filling the order, Pharmcorp must have immediately red-flagged it, and linked her name with the DP order. They usually weren't that efficient.

He ordered the medication with one of his code cards that he'd reported stolen months ago. Then he misdirected the theft report to take advantage of less-than-perfect networking between corporations. It was one of the several ruses he used to cover his work with Asher Wind Storm and Defy. Most of the time he got away with it; it usually bought him more time. But ordering the restricted stabilizer was beyond that kind of finagling; it begged for trouble.

He looked around the empty room and studied himself in the uninterrupted mirrored walls. His eyes were large saucers, filled with fear. They stared back at him like they weren't his own, more like those of an alien from another planet.

Being captured by the Aughts and the exhausting journey back to San Francorp had been traumatic. But having the CAPOs drag him here was way beyond that as a fear factor. He needed to rest. Instead, he was pushed to the edge of his endurance. He had no time to mentally prepare for an interrogation. He was worn down, drained, and close to collapse.

The surrounding reflections jumped out at him and made him feel entombed. He turned away and looked down through the transparent floor. He seemed to hang over a black void.

His stomach churned.

What time was it? He glanced at his bare wrist; fear turned to anger. They'd taken his watch, probably to heighten his sensory deprivation.

He hadn't yet been charged, or even questioned. Everything seemed out of sequence.

He understood the psychological torture of starkness and isolation, but knowing about it didn't seem to help him accept it. He felt helpless.

His shoulder nagged at him; the throbbing was hard to ignore. He wanted to massage the area, had to stop his hand from rubbing it. Storm had given him some mumbo-jumbo treatment that had no scientific grounding. As a neuroscientist he doubted its value, but there was no denying he hadn't been able to stand up prior to Storm's "healing."

He knew the CAPOs were watching behind the array of mirrors. Watching for weakness.

Watching for vulnerability.

Everything had to appear normal. He couldn't allow them to witness his pain. He might be able to field their questions about his wounds. Then again, maybe he couldn't. There was no doubt the wounds would be hard to explain. Better to try to act normal. Whatever that was.

Andrew took a deep breath, pushed his head back, stared at the ceiling. It was a mistake.

His splintered image bounced back at him from a crazy mosaic. The effect was nauseating.

He gripped the sides of the stool to steady himself, pulled his eyes away from the ceiling and pretended to yawn, then swallowed the burning bile that erupted into the back of his throat.

Isolation, exhaustion, and pain were eating him up.

He drew himself into an inner world, into the repetition of a silent chant, repeating the mantra he'd used since childhood. Its focus was the integral part of Valek's Mind Stimulation, a philosophy his parents—who were friends of the philosopher—practiced throughout their lives. Even though Andrew started learning the method as a child, it had taken most of his life to master the discipline.

Valek was a non-traditionalist who turned his back on accepted techniques of achieving tranquility by emptying the mind. Instead, he championed a method he called circuit breaking.

Overload the mind, push it into a frenzied delirium, then let everything go, slide into freefall.

Andrew visualized heat, shooting flames that spewed, filled every crevice of his being until volcanic lava flowed into a fiery pathway that seared, cauterized every neural circuit. All other incoming stimuli died. A bath of perspiration washed his body.

His mind had finally been released into freefall.

* * *

A seamless panel at mid-wall slid open. Emory Dutton walked into the room, accompanied by two CAPOs. The CEO ignored Andrew as he listened to someone on his telelink. Dutton frowned and impatiently jiggled the communicator clipped to his ear.

"You're disappointing me, Potek."

Dutton listened for a moment.

"I'll have more to say about this later, Commander. Much more."

Dutton clicked off the telelink and stood before Andrew, hands jammed into his pockets. "Do you know why you're here, Dr. Potter?" the CEO asked.

"I have no idea. Undoubtedly someone's made a huge mistake."

"What's your connection to Dr. Zoe Hidalga?"

"Zoe? She's an old friend; we went through medical school together." "And you've maintained that friendship?" Dutton said.

"I haven't seen her for a year or more."

"How close were you to her husband, Dr. Elliot Hidalga?"

"We were friends. I've been questioned previously concerning our relationship."

Dutton held up a hand and snapped his fingers. One of the CAPOs handed him a network file. He keyed through the contents, glancing up at Andrew every so often.

"Impressive!" He tapped the file thoughtfully. "Many of your robotic surgical innovations have gained worldwide recognition, from Moscorp to Riocorp."

Andrew nodded.

"And you've accomplished miracles with the CARE system."

Andrew waited for the axe to fall.

"I hope we haven't brought you along too rapidly." Dutton walked a circle around him, threw out another question. "Is Nathan Quinn an old friend also?"

"That's not a familiar name."

"I would think you would know the new head of Desisto Processing since you are actively involved with programming the CARE units."

"You're probably right, except no one seems to hold on to that job for very long."

Dutton's lips tightened. He thrust the computer file at one of the black-clad CAPOs. "You're here, in that seat, because your Ident-card was used today to order a restricted drug for Zoe Hidalga."

"Zoe?"

"Dr. Hidalga is a fugitive and your Ident-card was used to order X66 Recomb II. Explain that, please!"

"I can't; I haven't directly ordered medication for anyone in weeks, maybe months."

"Don't lie, Dr. Potter. The closed prescription authorizations report lists the prescriber as Medi-Prog number 03531. That *is* you, isn't it?"

"Not currently That card was reported stolen months ago. My code was changed to 228-A. You'd know that if you'd taken the time to do your homework."

Dutton turned his back on Andrew. "But an interesting coincidence, don't you think?" he shouted at the far wall. "Your stolen card used to order the restricted VMAS stabilizer for an old friend. A friend who's in trouble, I might add."

"I don't believe you. How was this diagnoses made? And if it's true, why is she still alive?"

"The woman was diagnosed via Noncorp CARE Unit #2 as having stage-three VMAS," Dutton said. "She went into the Noncorp sector for her diagnoses. And we both know she would have been disposed of by now if she went to a Corporit MD."

"But you say she's still alive and a fugitive?"

"To this point, she's eluded the CAPOs."

"But I can't believe Zoe would even enter the Noncorp area. Is there a border scan verifying this?"

Dutton face turned a bright red. "Don't concern yourself

with the obvious. Again, *your* stolen card authorized a stabilizer for Zoe Hidalga. That's not a coincidence that I can accept."

"Poor Zoe. It's not only sad to hear she has VMAS, but I can't imagine her as a fugitive for any reason. It's just so hard to believe. What's the charge?"

"She's diseased. That's the charge. And isn't that a ridiculous question from a someone with, I'm told, a brilliant mind. *You* programmed CARE, didn't you, Doctor?"

"Of course."

"Well, your huge mental capacity should be able to answer that question." Dutton sneered at Andrew. "That's why she's now on the DP list. And we will hunt her down and eliminate her, rid this diseased individual from our population."

"So that's why I'm here?"

"This is my party, not yours. I'll ask the questions."

"And I've been answering them. Charge me or release me."

"Not just yet, Doctor."

"Then I request representation from Advocatecorp."

Dutton looked at his watch and smiled. "We still have some time before I'm required to honor that request." He nodded to one of the security guards, who aimed an electronic stylus at the ceiling. An articulated arm with a tiny needle-like probe descended and hovered over Andrew. He felt a prickle of pain as the device entered his scalp.

"This whole thing's a farce, Dutton."

The CEO ignored him and grabbed the stylus from the CAPO, and pressed a button.

Andrew twitched; his mind lit up like a Christmas tree when the surge of electricity exploded inside his skull. Bursts of hot red and yellow lightning blinded him.

"That was just a biopsy to see if we need to operate," Dutton said, slowly circling him again.

Andrew's eyes followed the dancing dots of color; spittle ran down his chin; his pants were warm and wet. He wouldn't be taken by surprise again.

"I'll ask you one more time. What's your connection to Zoe

Hidalga?"

"I told you, she's an old—"

Dutton activated the stylus again. This time Andrew took command of the electrical charge, directing it along deadened neutral pathways until it dissipated harmlessly. Still, for Dutton's benefit, he let out a terrifying scream.

"What are you and Nathan Quinn involved in?"

He squeezed his eyes shut, forcing tears to flow. "I've…never … met…Nathan Quinn."

Andrew could feel Dutton's breath on his cheek as he forced Andrew's eyelids open. The CEO held his gaze for several seconds before he broke off the contact.

When Andrew opened his eyes, Dutton glanced at his watch.

"Unfortunately, I seem to have run out of time."

Chapter 28

Medi-Prog Complex
Robotics Unit

Valek's discipline was the only thing that kept Andrew Potter from limping as he left the CAPO transport. Hiding his pain was a battle fought with every step. The wounds from the Aught attack, CAPO interrogation, and sleep deprivation were bringing him down like a sinking ship.

He refused to count the hours since he'd slept. He was due in surgery right this minute.

Sleep was not an option.

Clashing with Emory Dutton had not only been painful, it had put him in the spotlight, a hair away from exposure. Dutton didn't have anything substantial yet or the interrogation would have been much more invasive. Andrew wasn't sure he could have withstood it. Not today.

This is going to tie my hands for a long time. That bastard Dutton will watch my every move now.

Andrew entered the Robotic Medical Facility, a gray, gloomy building that shot up to within a few feet of the city's covering dome. He nodded at the security cameras embedded in the ceiling as though it were any other day and placed an eye against the designated aperture for a retinal scan. After riding the elevator up to the surgical suite, he headed straight for the decontamination area.

At least no one will follow me in here.

He glanced at his watch, which the CAPOs had reluctantly returned upon his release from interrogation.

He was late.

Andrew casually looked around. Paranoia settled in; everyone seemed to be side glancing him. He wanted to lie down, to rest, but he knew any deviation from his routine could mean a death sentence, not only for him, but for his Defy cell and maybe even the entire network.

He should have ignored Zoe's death sentence. His knee-jerk reaction may have saved her life, but it had put him, and more importantly, the Defy organization, into the direct line of fire. From now on, he would have to be very careful. He couldn't afford to have Dutton and the CAPOs on his ass.

But he couldn't help it. Every time he tried to put Zoe out of his thoughts, he remembered the day they took Laya away to the orphanage. Zoe screamed and kicked as they tried to control her. Both grief for the loss of her husband and the wrenching away of her child overwhelmed her. Andrew had had to fight hard, pull in many favors to keep Psychcorp from neutralizing, deadening selective neural pathways to eliminate all the painful avenues that were making her unstable. But he'd sworn to Elliot that he would always be there for her.

After entering the chamber, the door snapped shut behind him with a loud whoosh of air. He immediately started stripping. When ready, he checked his sutured thigh and carefully rotated his shoulder. Things seemed unchanged. At least they weren't worse.

Andrew never enjoyed this part of surgical preparation, it was mostly an uncomfortable necessity that he had to repeat much too often in the last few days. The painful wounds the Aughts had given him would continue to threaten his life if they weren't constantly treated with care and medication.

With all this scrubbing, these damn wounds wouldn't dare have any microbes.

Ironically, the soft music in the units sometimes soothed him and allowed him to review each of the projects he was involved in. His left-sided brainpower had the natural tendency to create order, rivaling the very robots he'd designed. Each of his cybernetic creations always evolved into schematics that claimed an area of his cerebral storage. Like ancient filing cabinets, he could pull out each idea and view it whenever he was ready to redesign or work on it.

But since his wounds, his focus had turned to merely

surviving the preliminary decontamination preparation and getting through the day unnoticed. The development of new ideas would have to wait.

His superior logical abilities were discovered at the age of ten, when he designed his first robotic program. He'd replaced existing models with such impressive originality, Robotic Division paid for all of his costly cybernetic education.

Throughout the years, he improved every existing cyber surgical procedure. Brain and spinal injuries became his medical specialties. His robots had such fine-tuned skills, they were able to perform surgeries with a kind of accurate delicacy that made human hands seem clumsy and dangerous.

Today, as he stood in the steaming fumigation chamber, he leaned hard against the wall. Everything made him hurt, from the bactericidal-virucidal jet steam bath to the depilatory scrub. The warmth made his eyes go heavy; the stimulant he'd taken twenty minutes ago had barely kicked in, certainly not enough for him to notice any real change.

He forced his naked body through the exit into the operating area where he was gowned and gloved by a technician, who ignored his body wounds. She placed a helmet of tightly woven filaments on his head and hooked up dangling threads to the waiting robot.

"Your color today, Dr. Potter?" the surgi-tech asked.

"Light blue feels right."

The tech hit a button and the room's atmosphere softened to a blue glow that integrated with the walls. Andrew could still smell the residue of the fumigation and decontamination processes, but the air around him glowed as though he was in a blue fish tank.

A hologram of the patient's medical file appeared in front of him. He scanned through the history: twenty-year-old building jumper, the younger set's idiotic game of swinging from building to building using metal vines to propel themselves. This one misgauged, had slammed his head into a wall.

Trauma teams had managed to rescue and patch up most of

him, but his hearing was compromised; spoken words were a problem, along with short-term memory loss. He couldn't categorize objects. The file went on and on, but basically it was a typical right lobe injury.

The patient was the son of a Pharmcorp CEO, which was the only reason anyone was bothering with him. Otherwise, Desisto Processing would have finished him off.

Telemetry showed that the patient was surprisingly stable, except there was no brain activity in a portion of his right temporal lobe. Well, Andrew would give the young jerk his best effort. At the very least, he might learn something new.

"I assume he's hypothermic…you know I like them good and cool. If not, we might as well all walk out of here now," Andrew said, looking at an anesthetic tech.

"He's ready, Doctor," the tech said.

Andrew's self-administrated stimulant was finally having the desired effect, pushing Andrew's focus into super drive. Every piece of the procedure ahead became a visualized, detailed map in the synaptic-hook between him and the robot, Techton, who would actually perform the surgery.

Andrew would do the thinking.

"Techton, how are you today?" he asked the robot.

"I am fine, Dr. Potter. Quite ready to proceed." The cyborg's voice was no different in inflection or articulation than anyone else's in the room.

"And decontamination?"

"Accomplished twenty minutes ago," Techton said.

Smart aleck. Bawling me out for being late.

Andrew knew his thoughts would immediately be transmitted to Techton, but it wouldn't care. Its specialty was neurobiological interaction, not emotional nuance. And after all, what mattered most was that the cyborg performed the surgery exactly as Andrew transmitted to its neural centers.

* * *

Andrew returned to his office as though nothing had happened, ignoring the questioning stares of his staff. He assumed they'd had their own interrogations by the CAPOs. He refused to answer or acknowledge their probing remarks, not even those of his assistant, Tia. He intended to treat the rest of the day business-as-usual. He dropped down hard into his chair, upsetting its pneumatic balance. Annoyed, he tapped his fingers on the desk as he waited to regain equilibrium.

The idiotic jumper had not only survived surgery, he would probably be able to go swinging into walls. Again.

Youth really is wasted on the young.

More importantly, Andrew had earned the gratitude of the patient's powerful father, and that might come in handy one day.

He reached over and checked his electronic mail.

"Dr. Nathan Quinn requests a consult. Please call."

"Now there's a coincidence," he muttered to himself. "Or is that bastard Dutton continuing to play games with me?" He drummed his fingers on the desktop. Curiosity won out. He dialed Quinn's number.

"This is Andrew Potter in Robotics," he said when Nathan answered. "I have a message here to call you."

"Thanks for returning my call. I need some advice on robotic liver implant techniques, particularly in conjunction with imminent multi-organ failure."

"I don't understand."

"I realize you're a neuro specialist but I'd hoped to hear your thoughts on this one." "That's not the point. I wasn't aware that Desisto was involved in implants. Organ Harvest usually handles that end of things."

"This has to do with a clinical research project," Nathan said, obviously ignoring Andrew's sarcasm. "I'd appreciate discussing it with you in person."

When he didn't immediately respond, Nathan suggested: "Have you had lunch yet?"

"No, but I'm extremely busy and I've already lost the entire morning. Just tell me what you need to know."

"I need to show you some background material on the problem at hand. If not lunch, at least a cup of coffee? I'll only take ten or fifteen minutes of your time."

"All right. It's been pointed out to me that it's probably time I met the head honcho of Desisto anyway."

"Good! I'll meet you at the main entrance to the Medi-Prog cafe in five minutes."

Before Andrew could object, the line went dead. He shifted uneasily in his chair, staring at the silent telelink resting in his hand.

* * *

It was past the busiest part of the lunch hour and the dining area was emptying out. They had no trouble finding a table. While they waited for their order, Andrew studied the blond man sitting opposite him. His smooth, patrician features and his impeccable manners suggested that he was exactly what he claimed to be: a rich, privileged climber.

"There's no research project," Nathan said quietly "I need to talk to you about Zoe Hidalga. I saw your prescription order for the VMAS stabilizer."

"So?"

"You do know Dr. Hidalga, right?"

"Dr. Quinn, I just spent a most uncomfortable morning with Emory Dutton, who probably has already informed you that Zoe Hidalga is a friend."

"Zoe's my friend, too." Nathan frowned. "I have no direct connection with Dutton," he said. "In fact, I tried to warn you this morning that ordering X66 for her would put you at risk. Zoe is Desisto-listed. Obviously, I was too late."

Andrew hesitated while the waiter served their food. He had no appetite for the synthetic, tasteless pseudo hamburger, but rearranged it on the plate and took a bite. The whole day had an ironic twist: first the interrogation by Dutton, now this bizarre encounter with Nathan Quinn, all on the fifth anniversary of the day his entire life was turned upside-down.

* * *

Up until the day his parents died five years ago, Andrew's only interests were his education and career. Cybernetics was his passion and his incredible rise in Robotics had been easily accomplished by inventing innovative organ and body implant techniques. But when he unveiled his direct cybernetic-human interface, he was in the upper stratosphere of Corporit world recognition. Andrew's cybernetic patents generated incredible wealth for any venture capitalist or corporation that invested in his ideas. Calling Andrew a narcissist would have been a kind description.

In the midst of making funeral arrangements for his parents, he'd been notified that Advocatecorp was holding a registered communiqué, the confidentiality of which would be honored only for sixty days, as authorized under inter-Corporit agreement.

He let it go until the sixtieth day. But after picking up and signing for a sealed envelope, he found only a single micro storage device. He downloaded it to his computer, expecting to find some kind of statement settling his parents' estate, or even a personal note from them. Instead, he was stunned to learn that the death of his parents in a fire was not an accident. They had been warned and knew they were going to be deliberately terminated. That brought him crashing down to earth.

The words that flashed across his screen described their involvement in an underground movement that was working to overturn the Corporit structure. It was an indictment of Corporit culture and the path it had taken, a damning evaluation of a system that had put technological advancements ahead of human rights, and protection of the environment.

He was instructed to destroy any trace of the information for his own protection.

There was a final declaration of his parents' love for him, and a plea that he not only be understanding of their revolutionary activities, but find it within himself to carry on their work, not out of revenge, but because he recognized there was a desperate need for change.

They had given him a single contact: Asher Wind Storm.

* * *

Andrew suddenly realized that Nathan Quinn was waiting for him to pick up the conversation.

"What's your interest in Zoe?"

"As I've said, I'm a friend, just as you are. I was afraid she was lost when her name turned up for Desisto. Then when I saw your prescription order for her, I hoped—"

Andrew held up a silencing hand. "I've stuck my neck out for Zoe, but all I have is your word that you're a friend." He paused. "I've known her for years and never once heard her mention your name. And your current job in Desisto Processing doesn't exactly inspire confidence."

"What can I do, what can I say to convince you?" Nathan Quinn's eyes grew intense. "I could tell you how we grew up together, how she was my first love." He realized he was slumping and sat up taller in his chair. He hadn't meant to slip back into that earlier time.

"But that's still only my word," he continued. "If you feel you can't trust me, then leave. I'll find another way to help her by myself."

Andrew studied Nathan, thought about what he'd just said. He'd been trusting his intuition, and little else, for the past five years. He decided to take a chance.

"The problem is how to deliver the compound," Andrew said. After being interrogated by Emory Dutton this morning…well, I'm sorry to say I have to let Zoe's situation go. I simply have to lie low. The truth is, there's nothing more I personally can do to help her."

"But maybe I can," Nathan said.

"Maybe. But you need to know that Dutton's trying to piece together a puzzle that involves you, me, and Zoe. I don't think he's found the links yet, so this meeting needs to be as short as possible. And the last public one we ever have."

"You think the CAPOs are spying on you?" Nathan said.

"Without a doubt. And on you, too."

"Are you certain?"

Andrew gave him a wide smile. "I've already spotted two

of them watching us." He watched Quinn stifle the urge to look around.

"Any suggestions on how we handle this situation?"

Andrew took a tiny nibble of his burger. "I had a plan, but without me, it requires serious revision."

"Look," Nathan said. "I'll get the stabilizing compound to her."

"How?"

Nathan leaned forward across the table. "You get me the damn X66, tell me where to take it, and I'll find a way to get it to Zoe."

Andrew nodded. As they got up to leave, he moved in close to Nathan. "You better find some poor slob who really does need a multi-organ transplant for your so-called research project."

"Already covered."

Chapter 29

Cable Car Conglomerate
Corporit Singles Complex #2

After Andrew Potter left the cafe, Nathan faked total absorption in his handheld telelink while he tried to spot the CAPO that was supposed to be following him.

He saw nothing out of the ordinary.

Stalling, he pretended to place a few more calls. When the restaurant patrons thinned out even more, Nathan left the table and started walking toward the exit. It was then he spotted his tail, moving in a little too close, a little too rapidly, trying too hard to blend with a scattering of departing people. The man certainly wasn't a stereotype for the role, or was he? Slightly obese, dressed in brand new running gear, sneakers snowy white and unscuffed. Other than the ridiculous disguise, it was more the way he openly focused on Nathan.

Gotcha, you bastard.

At first, the thought of being shadowed created a certain weird excitement. Nathan's life had always been too *normal* and this gave him a sense of adventure far removed from anything that had ever happened to him.

It was fun to play-act.

Then reality hit him. He'd always been a person who did as he was told, followed directions. Protocol wasn't something he questioned. Mainly, he didn't like complications, avoided them whenever possible. Now, he was in way over his head and beginning to have second thoughts about ever getting involved in Zoe's dangerous situation.

At thirty-eight, his life had become predictable and comfortable, that is, until his appointment as chief of Desisto. This corporation was different than anything he'd ever been involved in, and the new job had brought nothing but doubt and second-guessing about everyone and everything, including his superiors.

He mapped his career path carefully. His family had made it plain from the time he was a child that he was privileged and influential, perhaps, even among the elite.

Old money. That is how his family referred to their situation.

Nathan had always resented being described that way. His mother and father devoted their lives to medicine, helping sick and suffering people, and they rarely ever talked about money. But they did talk about privilege.

With privilege comes responsibility.

That's what his father always said. But for the first time, Nathan was questioning where those responsibilities were going to take him.

The job as chief of Desisto Processing seemed like a perfect fit for him. The need for intelligent management, along with the concept of population control, could definitely be an extension of his statistical healthcare and delivery systems background. Outwardly, DP made sense, especially when food and other natural resources were now in such short supply. Without some kind of limitations and rationing, there would be chaos. But it never once occurred to him that Desisto might be used as a ploy to gain and retain power.

The past month had given him a new perspective. Desisto was not the manifestation of "the good death" or benevolent euthanasia, a concept that had seemed logical, and which made him comfortable with the program. But DP had been subverted to include the elimination of Corporit dissidents, political enemies, chronic complainers, Defys, and disruptive innovators. Now, its scope had expanded to include chronic illness and the elderly. Corporits and Noncorps.

He'd been a good citizen, stuck to the rules his parents promised would bring him continued wealth and happiness. But the threat to Zoe made it personal, made him question the whole system.

Nathan entered his apartment building and wanted to wave

good-bye to his watcher, who had been joined by another man also dressed in sports gear.

Two of them!

The pair stood across the street, pretending not to look his way. Instead of waving, he tucked his hands firmly into his pockets and stifled the temptation.

Safely inside his penthouse, he undressed quickly and stepped into the shower, allowed the hot steam to penetrate his pores and ease his tension. Afterward, he nestled into a robe and roamed through the apartment, reacquainting himself with the books in his library, dragging his fingertips across the piano keys. He started to sit down to play, but realized he was too restless to really concentrate on playing music.

The buzz of the lobby intercom disrupted his thoughts. The security robot wanted permission to allow Seka Joraine to use the vaculift.

* * *

Seka pressed down a fresh patch behind her ear and stepped into the lift. Although the sexual enhancer's aroma wasn't unpleasant, the thought of what it did, the powerful attraction it created, made her breathless.

Was this patch stronger than the others she'd used during the last two days? Probably not. She just hated wearing it at all.

Right from the beginning, right from the moment she stepped into Emory Dutton's office, it was all she could do not to back out of the assignment. She wasn't used to deceit, or living a lie, or having to pretend she was someone she wasn't.

Pretending?

Her feelings for Nathan were real. Even before she wore the enhancer, she was drawn to him. Would she, could she, do anything to hurt this man? She didn't know the answer. And Dutton was not only asking her to be someone she wasn't, he wanted her to be his personal spy. And if she didn't do what he requested?

She already knew the answer. And the thought of it made her shiver.

Maybe in some weird way the patch was affecting her, too. Maybe that's why her attraction had become so intense. She was at a point where she could barely stand to have Nathan out of her sight.

It wasn't supposed to work that way.

She looked into the lift's mirror and pushed a scatter of stray hairs into place. She wondered if Nathan would be happy to see her. Would he still want her?

Of course, you idiot. They don't call it chemical enhancement for nothing.

And if there was no patch?

* * *

"Hi, Seka," Nathan said when the lift door slid open.

They stared at each other: she at the threshold of the vaculift, he leaning against the polished wood apartment door. She couldn't help herself—her heart raced at the sight of him. It was obvious that he was not only surprised, but more than happy that she'd come.

"Hello, yourself," Seka said. "Are you going to ask me in?"

"I'm thinking about it."

"Well, while you're thinking about it, I'm going to get comfortable." She laughed and removed her full-length coat, posed for him in the nude.

Nathan took three long strides, looked up and down the hallway, and hurried her inside.

Seka could smell the pheromone enhancer in the air around her, but Nathan seemed unaware of the scent. He followed her into the apartment; she turned and rolled into his arms. Loosening the sash of his robe, she molded her body to his. Beads of perspiration erupted on his forehead. Seka looked at his flushed face, watched him struggle for air while his fingers tightened on her bare back, then slid down onto her hips. His arms and legs started shaking, first with tiny tremors, then with convulsive thrusts.

She slipped out of his arms and his hands curled into claws. He winced from the spasms—tendons bunching into rigid, knotted wires.

Nathan shoved her away.

"There's no air in here," he said, holding his twisted hands up in front of him. "I can't breathe."

"What's wrong?"

"I don't know." He stumbled toward the sofa. "I'm burning up, something's crushing my chest."

His color changed from bright red to a ghastly gray. After helping him onto the sofa, she reached behind her ear and yanked off the tiny transdermal patch.

"Let me get a damp cloth for your forehead." She hurried into the bathroom and flushed the chemical enhancer down the toilet. By the time she returned, Nathan's color had improved; his breathing was almost regular.

"Feeling better now?" she asked, wiping his face.

"Yes," he whispered. "I don't know what happened."

"Maybe you're allergic to me." She laughed nervously.

"God, I hope not!" He wiggled his fingers, which were flexible again, trailed a fingertip down her neck and across her shoulder. He pulled her onto the sofa next to him. "Just happened to be in the neighborhood, huh?"

"What?" Seka's mind spun in fear. She'd almost killed him! "I wasn't expecting to see you tonight."

Tears welled in her eyes.

"Hey, what's going on?" Nathan said. "We hardly know each other and I'm making you cry already?"

"I was so worried about you."

"I'm fine now." He took the washcloth from her and dabbed at her tears. "How about some wine?"

"No, I think I'll pass on the wine. But I'd love a cup of real coffee." When he started to rise, she pushed him back. "Tell me where to find everything."

Before returning to the living room with their coffee, she paused in the large formal dining room and unwound a filament transmitter from her little finger. She was confused, her mind racing in every direction.

She didn't want to hurt Nathan, but there was no way she was ever going back to Organ Harvesting, no matter how she felt about him.

She twisted the bugging device onto the stem of a silk flower displayed in a tourmaline bud vase, made sure it was really invisible. The bug would continue to pick up their conversation for Dutton's surveillance team.

For the next three hours, the two of them listened to and discussed music. She was a fan of the ancients and adored the three Bs—Bach, Beethoven, and Brahms. He also enjoyed the ancients, but preferred the moderns—Ulal, Rolfe Z, Lukinski, and the latest prodigy, Clifford Alden, whose preludes Nathan often played on his concert grand. When the last symphony came to a crashing climax, he leaned back and stared thoughtfully at the ceiling.

"Why so quiet?" she asked, laying her head in his lap.

"I was thinking about the Organ Harvesting Unit. I can't imagine what it would be like to work day after day in that kind of environment."

"It was pretty horrible," she said, caught off guard.

"I've never been there. I guess there are a lot of other places I should have visited," Nathan said. "Recently, I've begun to look at things from a closer perspective. Things seem different, somehow."

"Research is the basis for future medical treatments," Seka said. "I really believe transplantation and implantation are taking us closer and closer toward immortality."

"Who wants to live forever?" Nathan said with a laugh.

"I do!"

"Yeah, well, tell me more about how that immortality department operates. What did you do there?"

"I was involved in the removal and preservation of major blood vessels," she said. "What kind of daily output are we talking about?"

She knew, but wasn't about to tell him. "I don't think I ever saw any statistical information on the unit's production."

"Did the hospitals supply you with sufficient bodies?" "There was never a shortage."

"Really? That surprises me. I guess we've become so specialized it's difficult to comprehend how Medicorp works as a total entity."

"Like everything else in the Corporit system," she said. "Separate, but interrelated."

"Shit!" he said, wiping his face with his hand. "Everything *is* interrelated. Desisto must be a major reason why there's never a shortage of body input for harvesting."

"I don't follow you."

"You've jumped from the frying pan into the fire, from receiver to supplier."

Oh, my God I can't let him go on like this.

It was either Nathan or Dutton.

She shuddered at the thought of being sent back to her old job, maybe even something worse, but she sat up and clamped a hand over his mouth. Placing a finger to her lips, she reached for a marker from her purse, scribbled a note on the palm of her hand. *Say nothing.*

Nathan sat back, puzzled. She took his arm and led him to the dining room and pointed to the hidden microphone.

When they returned to the living room, Nathan stared at her, stunned. "I think I should go," she said. "Tomorrow's a work day."

"It is getting late," he agreed woodenly.

"Are you all right now?" When he didn't respond, she added, "I could stay, if you like."

Nathan picked up her coat and purse, handed them to her, started toward the door, then stopped and shook his head. He said nothing, but after a moment, he took her hand.

"Stay," he whispered.

Chapter 30

Medi-Prog Building

Emory Dutton liked to wander through the deserted Medi-Prog administration building after hours. Every office, every cubicle was empty, quiet, a little eerie. And with the subdued lighting and dark shadows, it was as if he was not only invisible, but omnipotent.

He imagined himself sliding through walls like a faceless ghost, an all-knowing specter who could search the offices of not only the people he out-and-out distrusted, but also those who simply displeased him. There were many in both categories.

No information, no secret was out of his reach.

Ever.

He rummaged, studied, and one way or another, always found each person's secret hiding place.

Always.

And if he didn't like what he found, they were gone…instantly. Poof!

There were professionals who could do this kind of undercover work, and they were better trained than he was. He often wondered why he did it, and the answer was always the same.

Because he could.

The survivors in his corporation learned early on that there were no secrets from the CEO of Medicorp. Every medical procedure, every treatment innovation, every decision, had to have his stamp of approval or it went nowhere… except down the drain.

His peers often asked how he slept nights, and would remind him that the CEOs of the top three giant corporations—Agricorp, Energycorp, Pharmcorp—had revealed that insomnia was their biggest personal problem. Every single one of them worried about rebellious personnel and the overambitious employees who wanted to replace them.

But Dutton had no problem there; he damned well knew at all times what his employees were up to. No surprises in *his* corporation. Why would he sleep poorly?

Tonight, he was in Nathan Quinn's office, rummaging through the DP chief's files. The man had been on the job for over a month and he was still an unknown quantity. Dutton didn't like "X" people in his equations for success.

"X" equaled an unknown.

Desisto was not only critical, it was integral to his vision for the entire system. He needed the right person for Desisto. It was at the core of all his future plans; his legacy. Yet, nothing seemed to bring him the right candidate. Where were those who could see the big picture?

Not enough Duttons in the world.

Everyone he placed as head of Desisto sooner or later asked too many questions. As a result, they all failed his strict parameters. Now, he was stuck with choosing from wealthy or successful families and dangling the carrot of success in front of them, along with incredible amounts of money. The potential rewards always brought out the candidates. All unsuccessful ones…thus far.

And dead losers tell no tales.

He slid into Quinn's desk chair, leaned back, and looked at the ceiling.

Legacy?

Where had the years gone? He couldn't stop thinking about his sixtieth birthday…the day he would have to step down.

How many hours had he spent scrolling through Corporit law, searching for a back door to the dictum that he must retire at age sixty? He'd found nothing. Fact: on his sixtieth birthday he was out and his Board of Directors would appoint the next CEO. There was no reprieve.

Maybe he should have spent time grooming a replacement. But simply put, he knew that wouldn't change anything. He would still be out the door.

Thinking about it depressed him. The silence closed in and a sudden shiver gave him goose bumps. But he would have his legacy, no matter what. He would be remembered for controlling the population and eliminating virulent diseases. No one could take that away from him.

He sat up, tapped the necessary keys to enter Nathan Quinn's communication system. It came alive and filled the screen in front of him. He keyed in his special, private password for Desisto. Its entire history—successes and failures—flashed in front of his eyes, page after page.

Certain names stood out: Larry Yamamoto, Harrolia Lucke, Marda Singer, Daniel Trist, Martin Yeninas. Each of them had been in charge of Desisto, all brought to him through family connections. Families looking for a cushy, secure spot to tuck away a loved one, or, too often, a problem child.

But Emory Dutton didn't deal in safe, he dealt in success. Every last one of these *connected* people failed to perform as head of Desisto to Dutton's specifications.

Every one of them had disappeared.

Their families?

Not too many complaints there. They knew the score going in—life was short, and it could become even shorter if the family member gave Dutton any serious trouble.

When Dutton was on the rise, he'd had to claw his way to the top of the heap. There was no easy pathway to success then.

Things had been chaotic. Governments all over the globe were in a state of flux. Forests, crops, and vegetation were rapidly dying off; fresh food was disappearing.

Corporations united. As a vital force, they bought up stocks, infiltrated corrupt systems, and when each country fell—one domino after another—they were able to control every entity throughout the entire globe.

In the end, Corporit had bloodlessly deposed all the world's governments, ruling bodies that, through neglect or intentionally, had created a catastrophic milieu of global warming, famine, and overpopulation.

Many in the world charged that the Corporit takeover was a long-planned, carefully plotted conspiracy.

Not a conspiracy, according to Dutton and many others, but a product of good planning.

He tapped into the most recent logs of Nathan Quinn's communications as chief of DP, and scrolled through screen after screen.

Nothing after hours, no anomalies, no red flags; nothing but routine, DP-related communiqués.

And there was nothing mentioning Andrew Potter in any way.

Still, Dutton felt that tickle on his neck again. He just *knew* that somehow the two men were somehow connected. Reviewing Quinn's workload wasn't really telling Dutton what he needed to know.

Could Nathan Quinn, of the famous Quinn family, really handle DP? Could he do the job?

Dutton leaned back into the desk chair and thought of Nathan's parents.

Just their names—Rebecca and Tris Quinn—gave him an uncomfortable chill. In the early days, the two of them had fought against every single innovative idea Dutton had.

Population control? They were resistant.

VMAS termination? They objected.

Innovative organ retrieval and selective implantation? They were opposed—adamantly.

Had they truly expected absolute humane treatment in a dying world?

Apparently, so that's the kind of picture Dutton provided the Quinns, and all the other do-gooders. He revealed only those parts of the picture they expected and wanted to see…the parts they could handle.

From then on, Dutton was able to win over the Corporit National Council.

And the Quinns? They knew nothing of the realities of DP and VMAS control. All they were aware of were the numbers—

statistical digits. And Dutton made sure they never knew all the details that made those numbers work.

It had been an unbelievable revelation when Dutton learned that Nathan Quinn was pulling strings to become the head honcho at Desisto Processing.

Dutton initially suspected it was some kind of Quinn plot to undermine his authority, to get rid of him.

But Nathan had acted independently, vying for a position that he believed would allow him to help dying people receive the aid, comfort, and care they needed. He had not involved his parents.

Why?

Dutton pondered that question a long time. He concluded that there was some kind of riff between parents and son.

He had intended to turn Nathan down. Then it came to him that this could be a pathway to destroying the Quinns' reputations, discrediting them once and for all. And what better way to wound them than through their only son?

After that, he made sure Nathan was chosen for the position. And he intended to watch the younger Quinn very, very carefully.

But the weapons he sought eluded him.

Who, exactly, was Nathan Quinn? Was he like his parents? Or was he a mutation? Would he do what needed to be done once he discovered the truth about DP? Most important of all, was he a man Dutton could manipulate?

Nothing in the computer was giving him the answers he needed, one way or another.

Dutton had to arrange for a closer, more personal examination of the man. Maybe it was time to bring Potek into the equation. Desisto was too important to take any chances. Too much was at stake.

He tapped into the VMAS statistics. Things were getting worse and worse. It was beyond him why all the brilliant minds studying this plague couldn't produce a biological cure to wipe it out. Well, there were other avenues to follow.

Maybe a plague wasn't the worst thing that could happen.

* * *

Robotic Surgical Theater

Andrew called an emergency meeting of his Defy cell.

When *SURGICLONE SESSION* scrolled across the computer screens of the cell members, it brought them all to their usual meeting place at eight that evening.

Andrew went through the unbearable decontamination process yet another time. He dreaded the meeting, but he had to bring his Defy group up to date about his interrogation session with Emory Dutton. If anything happened to Andrew, the rebels would have to move quickly to protect themselves.

C said, "This constantly being fumigated hurts like hell. Those decontamination brushes are a bitch." He looked the others, each in turn. "See," he said. "A's thigh is oozing blood."

Andrew ignored the comment.

D was furious. "You know as well as I do that these additional meetings put us at terrific risk. Why are we here again so soon?"

"I was picked up by the CAPOs today," Andrew said, "and taken to their interrogation facility."

B's face flushed a bright red. "Why?"

"The pickup was ordered by Dutton."

"You haven't answered the question. Why?"

"I ordered a VMAS stabilizer for Zoe Hidalga."

"So you were brought to Dutton," D snapped, "because you helped Elliot Hidalga's wife? Is that right?"

"Yes."

"We've discussed this before. You agreed with us that you were sticking your neck out. You promised not to get involved again." D could barely contain his disgust. "But you did it anyway!"

B jumped in, "My god, that Dutton is a barbaric maniac." D remained silent.

"Look, I don't think there's anything to worry about,"

Andrew said. "It was a primary investigation. I think Dutton's interested in Nathan Quinn, the new chief of Desisto Processing, not me."

"Then why did he bring you in?" B asked. "That man doesn't do *anything* without a reason."

"He's overreaching. Trying like hell to get something on Quinn. He obviously wants to nail him. He's trying to put together some kind of connection between Zoe, Quinn, and me. He's only playing guessing games." Andrew held up a hand, eyed each of the other surgeons. "I know you're angry, but we've always agreed not to use people's names. We have to stop using real names right now."

Andrew's heart was pounding violently and his legs were starting to give out. Even the stimulants were becoming useless. If he didn't get real rest soon, his body would go into failure mode.

"No more names, agreed?" B said.

"In fact, let's just drop the whole damn thing," Andrew added. "It's over and done with."

They have a right to worry. I've put them all at risk by helping Zoe. Probably shouldn't have said anything about being questioned.

D's face was red and his eyes wild, but he said nothing. C and B were also visibly uncomfortable.

Andrew knew they were all thinking the same thing—if the CAPOs brought in any or all of them in an effort to uncover an active Defy cell, an automatic Class IV interrogation would be activated. They might all suffer brutal torture. And even though the results would only compromise three other people, that didn't matter much when the CAPOs were frying your brains…or any other part of your body.

But if Andrew was outed, that left only four other primary individuals who knew the real identities of the entire thousand plus Defy members.

And if I fold under interrogation, it could be the end of everything.

His fellow conspirators were becoming more and more agitated.

D shouted, “What’s the matter with you, A? You could have brought down the whole Defy movement…finished us all off!”

Andrew’s wounds burned with greater intensity; he was exhausted, near total collapse. He was unable to respond for a long moment.

Elliot, my dearest friend. Zoe, Zoe! I’m so sorry—our connection, any connection, is over.

“I promise it won’t happen again,” he said finally.

Chapter 31

Cable Car Conglomerate
Medi-Prog Complex

Nathan Quinn didn't want to be anywhere near his desk this morning. He was numb, disconnected, and lost in a whirlwind of emotions.

The corpcaf, with its heavy dose of caffeine, seemed to slosh in his stomach, had him jumping out of his skin, even if it did help him organize his thoughts and force him to focus on his computer.

He tried to project his mind into the computer. The all-seeing, all-knowing computer. A complex binary system that was supposed to be omnipotent with every possible answer buried deep inside; embedded in the guts of its core, its heart. Could this inanimate intelligence really tell him everything he needed to know? Did it have all the answers for the betterment of human existence?

The computer monitor stared back at him.

Questions and more questions. So many questions.

How could Zoe Hidalga, a friend from his distant past, jump back into is his life and manage to take up almost every moment of his thoughts?

How could Seka, a woman he'd trusted—was even in love with—spy on him?

Yes, spy on me.

She had to be a part of whatever was going on, otherwise she wouldn't have known about the listening device.

Yet she'd warned me. Why?

He looked at Seka and his neck tingled with tension. He stood, carried his cup with him, taking hurried sips as he walked around his desk and looked out through the glass partition so he could watch her. She was sitting at her computer; he could tell from the tilt of her head she was only pretending to work.

Damn! I want my old world back, a place where I can believe that things are good, things are right, that what I do is right.

Was compliance such a bad thing?

More questions.

Could he work in this Corporit power system and sanction murder? Could he stay, knowing the numbers he manipulated were not just theoretical exercises?

And could he ever feel safe again?

No. That feeling was never coming back.

Maybe he couldn't find all the answers, but he wouldn't let the questions distract him any longer. His mindless drifting would not keep him from doing what had to be done. No matter what it took or how dangerous it might be, he would get the stabilizer to Zoe. At least she was one person he could do something for.

He returned to his desk, dropped down into the seat, and concentrated on the data scrolling across the split-window information screen. He didn't dare miss Andrew Potter's coded message about the VMAS stabilizer. If he did, Zoe would die!

A knock at his office door jolted him back to the moment. It had to be Seka. He ignored it. He needed more time to think about her.

I can't talk now.

When the knock repeated, he hit the freeze key and spun around. "This isn't a good…" Emory Dutton stood in his doorway, not Seka.

"I came for the Aught data," the Medi-Prog CEO said, his eyes a stony gray. "I'm not interrupting anything important, am I?"

Words. Just words. And Nathan knew Dutton didn't care one way or the other.

"Uh, just the usual morning review," Nathan said, shifting in his chair. He needed to see what he had frozen on the screen. Instead, he reached out to lift up a gray, opaque carafe on his desk.

"Would you care for a cup of corpcaf?" he said, wondering if there was even any of the bitter-tasting synthetic brew left in the container. Dutton waved away the offer.

"Those Aught stats?" He held a hand out, expecting the information on a Doculate.

"They're being compiled," Nathan said, returning the carafe to its coaster. "You should have them on your desk sometime tomorrow."

"That will have to do, I suppose, but I'm not impressed with your performance, Doctor." Dutton closed in, stood next to Nathan and his desk.

"Is there something else?" Nathan asked, not daring to return to his scanning while Dutton was still in the room.

"Not really. I occasionally like to observe my people at work."

Nathan turned back to the screen. He knew his face flushed and he had to resist a sigh of relief when he saw only run-of-the-mill reports frozen mid-scroll on his screen. He tried to act natural, forced his shoulders to relax, certain the CEO was watching his every move. Sweat bubbled up under his armpits as he allowed the information flow to resume. No matter what happened, he couldn't miss the message from Andrew.

Dutton was so close he could hear him breathing. The depopulation numbers and other medical statistics rolled across the split fields while Nathan made meaningless notes about finding more efficient ways to coordinate medical services. It was the furthest thing from his mind, but he would play the busy executive, find a way to occupy his mind and ignore Dutton.

Andrew had not only planted seeds of distrust, it was being confirmed. Now, Nathan knew Andrew was right and he had reason to worry.

Then Seka had pushed the whole scenario to a new level by showing him the listening device in his apartment.

And this surprise visit by Dutton? Did this fit into the scheme of things? It had to. Nothing happened without Dutton's approval. If someone was spying on Nathan, the CEO was behind it.

More questions.

Why in hell would anyone want to spy on *him?*

It couldn't be because of Zoe. No one knew about their connection. Except Andrew Potter, and he had as much to lose as Nathan. Andrew was Zoe's friend, too.

Or was he?

All the answers pointed back to Seka. But how? Why?

Dutton was rummaging through a stack of papers at the edge of Nathan's desk.

Asshole.

Nathan glared at him. The CEO stared back for a moment, then went on to another pile of documents, barely missing a beat.

What the hell is he looking for?

He would have to trust Seka—especially after last night. A thrill settled in his groin, caught him off guard as he thought about her, about the two of them. They'd embraced, conscious of the bug that would record every sound, every single movement. At first, he'd been reluctant, but their silence created a sexual tension that swelled with every stifled murmur, every sigh. They finally ignored everything and surrendered to each other in wild abandon.

The message he'd been waiting for scrolled across the bottom of the monitor.

Quinn, Desisto.

Agree with research projections.

Potter, Robotics.

He wanted to smash down the delete button, but Dutton's eyes were following his every move and he knew the information would scroll again for one more circuit through the system. He had to get Dutton out of his office, even though he'd said nothing.

Must have missed seeing the Potter message...this time. Probably not the next time.

Nathan let the strip zip across the screen until that window went blank. Then he hit the intercom.

"Seka, please step into my office."

Dutton remained silent when Seka entered. He looked into her eyes for several beats, then left without further comment.

"What was that all about?" she asked, Nathan.

"I wish I knew."

* * *

Nathan hopped onto the ambulated walkway, tried to blend into the ebb and flow of the early lunchtime crowd. He found he wasn't accustomed to the push and shove of people on a limited time schedule. He was being jabbed and elbowed; at one point, he almost lost his footing. When he regained his equilibrium, he realized he'd almost zipped past the Pharmcorp outlet that he and Andrew had agreed to use. He ended up doing some pushing and shoving of his own to get off the fast-moving belt.

Inside the pharmacy, he acted casual, wandering from counter to counter, examining various items, rejecting some and placing them carefully back on the shelves, dropping others into his basket for purchase. Starting toward the exit, he tapped his forehead and headed directly back to the first aid section, where he examined the display of self-stick bandages. He found what he was looking for at the back of the shelf. A box with the manufacturer's name lightly underlined. He read the directions on the box…twice…barely nodded, and casually tossed it into his basket before walking to the checkout counter.

* * *

Seka stood outside the upscale Fast Step restaurant, searching every arriving face. The eating establishment was only a few doors from the office and it lived up to its name for quick service. When Nathan folded his hands around hers, she threw her arms around his neck and held onto him. Streams of people swirled around them.

"I missed you," he said.

"I was afraid you might not come."

"We need to talk." He took her arm and pulled her into the restaurant. Once seated, they both started to speak at the same time, words spilling out in a jumble.

They stopped, laughed.

"I'm a mess," Nathan said. "There seem to be spies everywhere. I don't know who to trust."

She squeezed his hand. "I swear you can trust me, Nathan."

"You'll never know how much I want to, Seka." He edged his chair around the table to sit closer to her. "This whole thing is confusing." He looked into her eyes. "For starters, how did you know my apartment was bugged?"

She was silent, then blurted, "You really don't get it, do you?"

"Isn't that what I just said?"

"Nathan, you're in charge of Desisto, the nucleus of Medi-Prog's population control. There are parts to this equation they'll never let you know about. They're worried about you, worried about what you will do when you see and comprehend the whole picture."

"Well, it's become pretty damn obvious that this isn't just any day job, or the usual step up the Corporit ladder that I thought it was."

"They have to know whether you'll cooperate with them, Nathan. They can't risk exposure."

Nathan threw his head back and laughed until the people at the next table looked up, their interest piqued. "That's what this is all about? Hell, why not just ask me? Of course, they won't like my answers."

"Nathan, pay attention. You're either with them…or you're dead."

"How do you know that?"

Seka studied the holographic waterfall cascading in the center of the room, its colored lights reflected on the artificial, airy spray. The noise level escalated as more and more people entered the popular café.

"Have you ever been inside the Organ Harvesting satellite?" she asked, her eyes mesmerized by the illusion of splashing water. "Don't bother to answer…I know you haven't."

The waiter interrupted. After he took their orders and

walked away, she continued. "People with privilege…people like you…don't have anything to do with Organ Harvesting. But for someone like me, it was the only way into medical school."

"How does that connect with Desisto and what's been happening to me?"

"Let me get to it in my own way," she said, looking away from the fountain image. "When I didn't make the medical school quota, I was offered entry into a special program. I jumped at it. It was my only chance. Ten years of servitude didn't seem important then. I would be a doctor."

"Ten is quick. Twelve is about what it takes any of us," he said.

"No, I'm talking about ten years *after* pre-med, med school, internship, and Organ Harvesting residency."

"Additional years?"

"Yes, ten years! And that isn't the worst of it. After you fulfill the contract, you still can't simply walk away. You have to obtain a special release. Some people spend their entire career in that department, always trying to transfer out. The unit has the highest suicide rate in Medicorp."

"But they finally offered you an opportunity to leave. Why?"

She placed her hands on either side of his face and held his cheeks. "Because I have a perfect biophysical match with someone they were interested in keeping tabs on. With a little chemical enhancement, I would not only be compatible, I would be sexually irresistible."

"You're the perfect biophysical match for…for…me?"

"Yes."

"Well, they sure as hell got that right."

"But in a way they never expected," she said. "I've fallen in love with you, Nathan." Seka gazed deep into his eyes. "All I had to do was cooperate and I was free."

"I'm sorry," he said, "but I'm glad we were thrown together. I can't imagine living without you."

"Maybe we can make Dutton think nothing has changed,"

Seka said. "Think I'm still working for him."

"So it *was* that bastard. I should have known."

"Of course it was Dutton. We all work for him." The waiter arrived, set their food down.

"There's something I must do," Nathan said after the waiter left. "After that, we'll find a way to get out of this…I promise … even if we have to make a run for it."

"But they're watching our every move."

"And we're watching theirs." He reached for her hand, held it. "We can do this." Then he told her everything about Zoe Hidalga.

Part 3

Chapter 32

Nathan stepped onto a deserted transpod station, the surrounding walls and floor covered by corporate advertisements. As he walked across the silent platform, his movement and presence activated a field of pop-up, life-sized holograms. The bright colors blinded him at first, then the blast of loud music startled him, making his heart boom in his chest.

Calm down. It's nothing.

He had no choice but to look at the largest of the pop-ups, an eight-foot-tall cosmetic hologram—a woman seated in front of a mirror, artfully applying Katie cosmetics. Past that, attractive models moved from provocative pose to provocative pose, wearing the latest in revealing evening dresses from House of Margee Fashions.

As he walked past a statuesque brunette in a see-through peasant blouse and slit-to-the- hip gaucho pants, he smiled, then laughed out loud. The ridiculousness of the encounter somehow quieted him. His mind kept creating continuous bizarre scenarios about his merging with each of the holograms, making love, and moving on.

He hadn't expected much pedestrian traffic in the transpod at this hour, and was right. The station was empty…except for one man, who had entered soon after Nathan arrived.

You've been on my ass all day.

The creep wore ridiculous warm-up sports gear, but Nathan had to admit the CAPO would probably blend well into any crowd with that getup. No one would give him a second thought. The phony jock spy stood at the opposite end of the platform, trying very hard not to look like he was watching Nathan.

No place to hide here, Jock.

Nathan was tired of being jacked around by people he knew nothing about. But then, he probably wouldn't have even known of their existence if it hadn't been for Andrew Potter, who'd told him about the nosy CAPOs.

In a flash of anger, Nathan sprinted over to the man and faced him, eye to eye. "What do you want?"

"Sir?" The CAPO was obviously thrown off guard. His mouth dropped open, his eyes blinked rapidly. "Hey, mister, I'm just waiting for the pod, same as you."

"Don't give me that bullshit. Who the hell are you working for?"

"You're making a mistake."

"Don't think so. You're part of Emory Dutton's crew, right?" Nathan grabbed the man by the upper part of his satiny jacket. "I don't like people following me, nipping at my heels. Got it?"

"I told you, I don't know what you're talking about." The man held his palms up in false surrender, but Nathan wasn't having any of it; he landed a hard punch to the center of the man's face. The loud crack told both of them that Nathan had shattered the nose of the CAPO, who crumpled to the platform, crying out in pain.

The transit pod pulled into the station, waited the required thirty seconds. Nathan slid through the door just before it clunked shut. At the window, he watched the man struggle to his feet, his face covered with blood. The CAPO pulled a telelink from his coat pocket, spoke into it. Their eyes held for an instant before the pod picked up speed and was gone.

* * *

Nathan knew every CAPO would now be on the lookout for him. He knew damn well he had to be especially careful to not be caught and hauled into a detainment center.

Should have tried to lose him, not bloody him. Hell, what do I know about this cloak and dagger stuff?

Nathan got off at the last stop, hoisted his backpack filled with extra clothes onto his shoulders, and slipped through one of the dome's sliding service doors into the open terrain. Others had come through here, but they were using the immediate outside area as a garbage dump. It took a while to get through the disgusting mess, but even then it was still stop and go. Roving border patrols kept him dropping to the ground and crawling on his belly for close to two hours.

The dense atmosphere was surprisingly clear, making the moonlight glow brighter than usual. At this point, his clothes were torn and his elbows and knees were bloody and raw from scampering over the sharp-edged rubble. Terrified, he kept checking his surroundings as he moved from shadow to shadow.

He paused to coordinate his surroundings with the map Andrew had enclosed in the bandage box that held the VMAS stabilizing compound. It was amazing that Pharmcorp could turn a year's supply of the valuable medication into something so feathery light. He'd examined the transdermal patches at his apartment and was impressed with the ingenuity that had created the lifesaving membrane. The patch would be completely invisible once it was applied.

Climbing over what he thought was the last huge mountain of debris, he thought of Zoe and the weird twist of fate that allowed him to see her name on the DP list when it scrolled across his computer monitor. She'd been black-flagged and he could still visualize the flashing DESISTO message that would have soon turned her into a statistic. He couldn't help but think what would have happened if his head had been turned away at the exact moment when her name came across his screen.

He put the memory out of his head and picked up speed. He was late and he hoped his connection was still waiting. Having come this far, he couldn't turn back. He would not abandon Zoe.

In his haste, he tripped over a mound of who-knew-what and sprawled on the ground. Something stabbed him in the thigh and without thinking, he screamed out angrily. He'd been pierced by a long, narrow shard of glass. Nathan clenched his teeth, hoped no one had heard his outcry, and listened for a long moment.

Nothing.

If he'd lanced an artery, pulling the dagger of glass out would probably kill him; he would bleed to death. But there was no choice. He was stuck in this deserted wasteland. Without letting himself think about it, he wrapped his handkerchief around one hand, held his breath, and quickly pulled out the shard. Only a trickle of blood darkened his pants.

He lay still, waiting for the pain and his pounding heart to settle, then turned and glanced over his shoulder. The lights of San Francorp were far away now, just a dim glow on the horizon.

Nathan envisioned Zoe as he'd last seen her as a teenager—tall, slender, long black curling hair, and dark inquisitive eyes. He'd fallen in love with her that summer at camp and they dated throughout high school. Then they drifted apart.

Yet, he was here because of her. She had become his wake-up call, the catalyst that had changed the way he looked at the Corporit medical system. And once he really did *see* it, there was no going back. Business as usual was out of the question.

His new job had turned him into an observer, a referee, a scorekeeper for the doomed, reduced to mere names flowing across his computer screen. These people had become the primary players in a complex Corporit game—Desisto, Monopoly, Scrabble, chess. The big difference with Desisto: death was always the winner.

Ahead, he saw the shadowy outline of a saw-toothed, decaying brick building, with two large circles propped on the top of one corner. That was his destination, provided he'd followed Andrew's map correctly.

Nathan was more tired than he'd ever been in his whole life; his mind kept drifting. An image of Seka flashed through his head. A rare, beautiful orchid with dewy skin, bathed in exotic scents. In his mind, her lips parted…

He shook away the vision and checked his bearings again, saw he'd drifted off course. Correcting his heading, he redirected his thoughts, yet Seka still remained with him, her face as vivid as if she were actually there.

Would she betray him?

A moving shadow separated from the large silhouette of the target structure. He whistled the opening notes of a Carrie ballad that Andrew and the others used as a code. He watched the figure edge closer. He whistled the strain again.

"God dammit, I heard you the first time!" a gravelly voice said.

"I just wanted to be sure," Nathan whispered, straining to see who was out there.

"Yeah, yeah! Where the hell have you been? I was about to leave."

"I'm being watched. I couldn't get here any sooner."

A craggy face popped up in front of him, looking startled. "And who the hell are you?" the man said. He pulled out a knife, waved it in the air.

Nathan jumped back, his eyes on the blade. "I'm Nathan Quinn. Andrew sent me."

A second figure ran toward them from a different building. The moonlight illuminated Zoe Hidalga's gaunt face.

"Zoe?" Nathan said.

She peered at him, then smiled and reached out to hug him. "Nathan Quinn! What are you doing here?"

"I've been wondering that myself for the past couple of hours."

"You know him?" the man said.

"Do I know him?" Zoe laughed. "Nathan and I spent many a moonlit night like this together, a long time ago."

"Where's Andrew?" the man asked.

Nathan told them how he and the doctor had met and how Dutton interrogated Andrew. There was no way he could have come.

"At the moment, Andrew's situation is more fragile than mine." He handed her the package of X66. "I've got to get back. Right now."

"Not without me," Zoe said.

Chapter 33

The Caplac Domes

Storm looked to the heavens, raised his hands to the moon. Ink-filled clouds rose higher and higher, swirled, then blocked the silvery glow.

He fought with the spirits within him, forces borne by his soul long, long ago when he was a child. Forces created to complete a mission.

And he'd followed that unfolding. Followed that chosen pathway with focus and purpose.

Until now. Now, he was distracted, torn.

With agitation, he lifted, flew with the wind. Up, up. His amber eyes searched the world below and found only blackness, emptiness.

Everything was closing in, smothering him, bringing him down.

He collapsed back, felt pain, the crush of terror in his heart.

Where was she?

I can't see her. I can't sense her. I can't feel her being.

Gone!

Her essence was not here with him.

It was gone.

* * *

Moonlight spilled through the high transparent dome, created a pathway of light that Storm followed as he paced back and forth in his quarters. Every few moments he stopped to touch the book of poems Zoe had held, as if that contact alone would bring her back.

There was so much he wanted to say to her. So much he needed to tell her.

From their first moment, when he touched her hand, he knew his loneliness was in the past. Behind him. He had found the one.

The gray wolf was nearby, wary, uneasy, resting on his haunches, but always ready to spring. His eyes tracked Storm's every step.

"I should have stopped her from going," he shouted at the wolf. The animal's fur bristled and it tilted its head, pointed both ears toward Storm.

He'd agreed to her going to see Andrew, who was bringing the medication. Now, she was long overdue.

She was gone. Swallowed up.

And he was angry at himself for caring too much.

"There's no time for this," Storm said to the wolf. He paced again. "Falling in love?

There's too much to be done. Do you hear me?" The wolf's eyes blinked back at him.

Storm turned to stare at the glowing moon.

"Andrew, what have you done to me? Why did you do this to me?"

It had only been a simple, ordinary request from Andrew, his closest collaborator. Rescue the woman. Save Zoe Hidalga, a Corporit victim. But from the start, he'd let his guard down, allowed himself to be drawn into her sphere, mingle with her essence, her being, her needs.

Yes, he had allowed it happen.

And now all he could think about was her. He would not rest until she returned.

* * *

The pounding at the door broke Storm's reverie. Man and wolf loped to the entry. "Jacob, where have you been? Where is Zoe? I trusted you—you and no one else—with that woman's life."

"Gone!" Jacob almost swallowed the word. He handed Storm a folded piece of paper. "She sent this."

He opened the note.

Storm, forgive me. I couldn't wait. I have to go for Laya now.

Zoe

"I couldn't stop her," Jacob said, unable to return Storm's piercing stare.

"*I* should have stopped her, stopped her from going to see Andrew."

"Andrew never came."

"What!"

"She knew the man. Called him Nathan Quinn."

"I don't know this man. And you were told to take her to Andrew only, so she could talk to him, assure her of his recovery. No one else, Jacob. No one else."

Storm felt his fury building, expanding, a force of nature that could explode into a crushing power of destruction. His mother had taught him to control his anger. Step by step, to restrain and master his massive power, to keep it from hurting others. Many had been injured when he was an untrained child. But he had learned and became the master of his abilities. And it had not come easy.

He looked away from Jacob and forced himself to slowly caress the wolf's fur. "Nathan Quinn said Andrew was under surveillance."

"Did this man bring the medication?"

"Yes."

The wolf's hackles settled.

"Thank you. I know you did your best, Jacob." The man flushed, nodded before turning to leave.

After the door closed, Storm sank to the floor. The gray wolf laid its head in his lap. "We'll bring her back," he said, stroking the animal's coarse fur over and over.

Chapter 34

San Francorp
Medi-Prog Headquarters

Emory Dutton leaned into a chair he'd deliberately placed far forward and exactly in the middle of the wide auditorium stage. The meeting hall was huge, but the seats were narrow, and everyone was cramped and uncomfortable in their restricted personal spaces. It was a no- nonsense gathering place, designed to hold a large number of Medi-Prog staff. And it was rarely used.

Dutton took in the perplexed expressions of the already seated staff, then turned his attention to those who continued to file into the auditorium. The room resonated with the loud buzz of conversation, undoubtedly about the unscheduled meeting.

He fussed with the communicator lodged in his ear canal. It had been slipping and sliding, driving him crazy for days; the promised replacement was back-ordered for weeks.

Weeks!

When he ordered something, he got what he wanted, usually in record time. Subordinate Corporit personnel usually made it their business to stay on his good side…his right side.

I'm going to have the head of the manager that markets these gadgets. My smart-ass nephew could do a better job with one eye closed.

He drummed his fingers on his thigh.

That's a damn good idea! Maybe that would get my sister off my back. She's been nudging me for months to find a slot for that young idiot son of hers.

He pulled out his memory unit and punched in a reminder to take care of it ASAP.

He couldn't leave his ear alone. He jiggled a fingertip inside it again, hoping to finally stabilize the ill-fitting communicator, but he knew that wasn't going to happen. It would only wedge itself into the wrong position again.

His other hand covered his eyes to conceal his annoyance, but he peeked between his fingers to read through a wad of memos in his notebook, sent through CAPO Communications Control early this morning:

> NATHAN QUINN WHEREABOUTS UNKNOWN. ASSAULTED AN OFFICER. ELUDED SURVEILLANCE.

The base of his spine tingled.

What's that son-of-a-bitch up to, dammit?

He'd hoped against hope that he'd finally found the right person to head Desisto. And a Quinn family rebel, to boot.

All he really wanted, and needed, was a competent, malleable manager. Against all odds, he'd found Quinn and hoped he would turn into an ask-no-questions hatchet man.

Dutton's assessment as to why Quinn took the job was that he wanted to strike out on his own, step away from the binding burden of the Quinn legacy.

But right now it wasn't looking good. In fact, he was beginning to think that Nathan Quinn would follow in the footsteps of all his DP predecessors—in the ring, then quickly down for the count.

Dutton punched in further notes to himself:

> LOCATE QUINN — MAXIMUM EFFORT ON HIS SURVEILLANCE INTERROGATE FINALIZE!

A loose cannon in Desisto could level the whole medical complex, along with his corporation, in a wild domino effect. In fact, it could rock the entire Corporit structure. The CNC took a long time to fully trust him. And they relied on certain Corporit secrets to remain that way—secret.

His heart thumped an extra beat.

Then, there was his Board of Directors. They weren't going to be very happy with another failed Desisto chief. And the worst of it all, it would make Dutton look weak and inefficient.

When the auditorium was almost full, he searched the rows, looking for Nathan Quinn.

Where the hell is that bastard?

Dutton would damn well have an answer. And soon.

He abruptly stood and walked with brisk steps to the podium.

"Ladies and gentlemen!" He waited a few beats, even beyond the point when the room became silent, to speak again.

"This is probably the most exciting day of my Medicorp career. At this moment, none of you can realize what a truly auspicious occasion this is. So I won't keep you waiting another minute."

But he did.

He kept them on the edge of their seats as he dramatically stared at staff members in each of the designated seating sections.

Finally, when virtually everyone was squirming and looking from side to side, he said, "It gives me great pleasure to tell you that we have made a significant medical breakthrough."

He paused again, soaking in the buzz of excitement that swept throughout the auditorium. Then he blurted, "We now, finally, have an effective vaccine for the Viral Mal-

Absorption Syndrome. It's approved for immediate general distribution."

It took a beat for the reaction to set in, but when it did, the entire Medicorp staff stood and the room shook with their applause, cheers, and whistles.

Dutton allowed the outburst to continue for several seconds before he raised both hands for silence.

"Incredible as it is, you need to understand that the vaccine is only effective on those who have never contracted the virus. But there is every indication that R&D will soon be successful in finding an all-encompassing cure for a disease that has so drastically infiltrated and caused so much suffering and death within the population."

Again, wild applause.

"In the meantime, we will be dramatically expanding production and distribution of a previously restricted VMAS stabilizer, X66 Recomb II."

Another round of approval.

It took a dozen of Dutton's half-hearted pleas for silence before he quieted the crowd. "Now, let's take a look at some of the immediate effects of this wonderful development.

Foremost, Organ Harvesting will have fewer problems treating and preserving organs infected with VMAS."

* * *

Dutton let his eyes roll past his watch. He had been speaking for more than an hour, delving into the intricacies of distribution. Usually, at these long general meetings, there were coughs, throat rumblings, and even a few yawns here and there. Not this time. Today, he had yet to lose the attention of a single person in the audience; the air crackled with excitement.

"And finally," Dutton said, looking up from his text. "For those of you who have petitioned repeatedly for improved Noncorp care, I'm pleased to announce that we will also vaccinate uninfected Noncorps, and distribute X66 to the infected population through the CARE units, starting sometime within the next three days."

The explosion of applause was deafening.

* * *

As the auditorium cleared, Dutton went directly to an adjoining conference room to meet with his senior Medi-Prog section chiefs. The dozen or so men and women were already seated around the conference table when he entered. Several called out congratulations. Dutton gave them a practiced smile and took his seat at the head of the table.

His eyes settled on Nathan Quinn. Where had the man disappeared to last night? "Dr. Quinn! How nice that you've decided to join us."

"I didn't miss any of it. I came in just after you started speaking. I sat in the back so I wouldn't disturb the others. Fantastic news."

Dutton wanted to point to the door; toss him out on his ass. Sharing confidential information with the man was risky. But there would be many complications if he arbitrarily fired him. He would have to deal with Dr. Quinn in private. There were many questions…and he would have the answers. Or else.

Dutton raised a hand for attention but spoke without waiting.

What you heard in the auditorium today is only a small part of the equation. And under no circumstances can any of you reveal what I am about to tell you."

Dutton stared at Nathan.

"If there is even a *hint* that one of you has leaked this information, that individual is as good as *gone.* Any questions thus far?"

Dutton watched their faces become distrustful. The initial atmosphere of good humor evaporated. Expressions ranged from quizzical to grim.

"The complicated task of monitoring population growth has been under our control for the last two years, but the Board of Directors of the Corporit National Council has voted to augment our measures. Despite extensive synthesis and numerous promising agricultural regeneration projects, the earth still remains incapable of supporting our growing population."

"What I'm about to tell you will directly conflict with the earlier announcement about the VMAS vaccine and stabilizer, but this is an overriding directive, and it's for department heads only.

"That directive is to *expand* Desisto Processing."

"I thought," Andrew Potter interrupted, raising his voice, "that Desisto was supposed to be a temporary expedient."

A low, angry buzzing vibrated throughout the room. Many nodded, mouthing agreeing comments.

Dutton bristled at the question. "There'll be time enough

for your input when I'm finished, Dr. Potter." He turned to study Nathan Quinn's reaction, but found only an attentive, impassive face.

Where did you go last night, you traitor?

"My comments about the vaccine remain accurate, but as of yesterday, the stabilizing compound...X66...has been reformulated to—"

Dutton had intended to soften the news. Instead, he blurted the revelation. "—to become an accelerator."

The gasps were audible, as though the air had suddenly become toxic. Everyone around the conference table first stared at him, then at each other.

"But that makes us liars and cheaters to the very people we're supposed to protect," the Pediatric Medi-Prog chief shouted. "It's murder, that's what it is!"

"You can't handle that?" Dutton countered. He waited impatiently, tapping his fingers on the tabletop.

"It seems...draconian," the head of Women's Health said.

"Not in the Darwinian sense. We have entered into the final phase—survival of the fittest."

"How is the accelerator to be administered?" said the senior Medi-Prog chief in charge of Poison and Disease Control.

"The same as we currently administer X66," Dutton said. "By transdermal patch."

"And the patients will think they're receiving a stabilizer, is that correct?" another asked. "We are really going to *lie* to them?"

"Yes!" Dutton said. "The plan is to create a mass, simultaneous distribution in both Corporit and Noncorp areas. All patients with VMAS will receive it."

"There must be something else we can do," the Pediatric Medi-Prog chief said. "Think of all the children."

Dutton knew he had to stop them now. Senior Medi-Progs had to face the grim reality of exactly where the future of the earth stood, once and for all.

"Do you think this is what any of us wants?" Dutton said.

"Let me assure you, it is not!

But the altered stabilizer is the most appropriate and economical way to rid ourselves of this diseased segment of our population. And together with the vaccine, we will not only rid our existing population of VMAS, but bring humanity's numbers closer to what our planet can sustain."

The silence was thunderous.

Chapter 35

San Francorp
Corporit Boarding School #3

The return trip had been exhausting and although Nathan tried to slow down for Zoe as often as possible, she kept falling back. Still, she kept pushing hard, pushing beyond her endurance. There was no turning back. It was a matter of either keeping up or being left behind.

By dawn, they'd barely reached the outskirts of San Francorp where they said their good- byes. Zoe quickly changed into clothes that had survived the rough trip in a plastin bag tied to her leg.

Ever watchful, she blended into the transpod crowds of people on their way to work and school. She used the travel pass Nathan had given her and headed straight for Laya's school.

Zoe walked slowly through the now deserted Syn-Park across the street from the orphanage and tried to pretend she was a casual stroller killing time. That kind of action in itself was a suspicious anomaly. Her teeth clenched as she waited for the CAPOs to appear and drag her away. But she held herself together and tried to pretend that everything was fine. She barely managed to keep from bolting out of the park.

She glanced across the street at her daughter's boarding school and eased onto a bench. Her peripheral vision took in the contours of the school's basic construction. It was a simple, large rectangle, created from ugly slabs of gray, composite stone. She could see no alternate entrance to the building other than the double doors at the front of the structure.

It was unbearable to think her beautiful child had spent two years inside this sterile institution with hundreds of other orphans. Had they been forcibly taken from their parents, too?

Zoe turned her attention away from the school and concentrated on scanning the artificial park foliage surrounding her.

It only added to her sense of alienation.

None of these unmarred, shining green, perfectly formed bushes or uniform multi-colored flowers came close to looking real or natural. They were more like the diorama props she'd seen at the Natural Museum of History, surrounding the extinct species of animals staring into space with glassy, dead eyes. If these plants had eyes, they would be just as lifeless, with none of the vitality of the living vegetation in Storm's Caplac domes.

Tears of frustration clouded her vision; a wave of dizziness left her breathless. Her fingers slid across her shoulder to the VMAS stabilizer patch that was now an enmeshed part of her skin. It wasn't helping her. If anything, she felt worse. She reached into her pocket for another neurostimulator and choked it down without any water.

Brushing hard at the dust on her dark pants, she pressed down on the multiple wrinkles as though that would iron them away. She'd found the outfit hidden in a corner of Arina's closet. It was the only piece of clothing the artist owned that even came close to the Corporit's usual severe tailoring and bland colors. It was chancy, though. If anyone gave more than a passing glance, they would know she was not dressed within Corporit standards and might wonder why and report her.

A shiver stopped her.

What have I done! I should have waited, listened to Andrew.

Like a fool, she'd avoided thinking about the specifics of rescuing her daughter, only that she had to take some kind of action to save her.

Stupid, stupid! VMAS must have turned my brain to mush.

Explosions of useless scenarios flashed through her head. The longer she sat, the weaker, the more uncertain she became. Alone, exposed, sitting in the Syn-Park doing nothing, was almost as dangerous as doing the wrong thing.

Right now, every CAPO must have a holo-image of her. The fact that they weren't already surrounding the school gave her a glimmer of hope.

Move! Move now!

A lone jogger dressed in sports gear hurried toward her. She tensed as he crossed the pseudo-turf and moved between the artificial trees. He held his distance and didn't seem to be looking at her. Still, there was something wrong about him. Or maybe she was just worrying about anything and everything.

Move! Get up! Go!

Her mind burst into hyper-drive as fragments of a scheme fired her. She would let the details fill in as she got into it. She checked the location of the jogger; he seemed to be taking a break, settled down on a bench, engrossed in an electronic reader.

She suddenly felt terrible. Beads of perspiration popped out, ran down her forehead; she braced for the expected gut spasms. But as quickly as the attack came, it was gone.

She tried not to hold her breath as she walked directly to a telebox communicator and used one of the tokens Nathan had given her. She punched a number into the telelink, her trembling fingers slipping twice before she got the correct sequence. Waiting for someone to answer, her legs started shaking; she could barely hold onto the receiver. Then someone answered.

"District School three, Nima Harper speaking."

"Harper, this is Captain Lear from CAPO Juvenile," Zoe said harshly.

"Who?"

"Pay attention. I said Lear, Juvenile."

"Uh, what can I do for you, Captain?"

"We're moving Corporit boarder Laya Hidalga into protective custody."

"Protective custody? Is that necessary?"

"Did I say this was a request? This order comes from Corporit HQ. Matron Castle will be arriving in two minutes to collect the child. Have her ready. Immediately!"

"But—"

"Matron Castle will explain when she arrives."

Zoe disconnected, tried to contain herself as she waited, drawing out the minutes. When she thought enough time had passed, she walked purposely across the street. The stainless steel security door looked substandard to Zoe. She was certain that someone with the right tools and skills could easily defeat the locking system. It seemed obvious they weren't worried about anyone stealing unwanted children.

She activated the electronic announcer and continued to study the surface of the metal door as she waited for a response. Under her breath, she rehearsed her impromptu role, trying to look as officious as possible. She clenched and unclenched her fists to work up the courage to do what had to be done.

The electronic lock clicked; the door swung open. A small woman dressed in a simple blue and white Corporit teaching uniform looked up at Zoe. Behind her, Laya sat on a straight-back chair, feigning interest in a book resting on her knees.

"I'm Matron Castle," Zoe said, stepping inside and closing the door behind her. She looked past the teacher. "I've come for the Hidalga child. Is that her?"

Laya's head jerked up at the sound of her mother's voice, but before she could say or do anything, Zoe checked her daughter with a warning glance.

"We'll need the proper authorization papers," the teacher said, eyeing Zoe's clothes with suspicion.

"I have them here," Zoe replied evenly, shoving her hand into her pocket. She coiled her hand around a roll of metal slugs, pulled out the reinforced fist, and slammed it into the startled teacher's face. The woman sank to the floor, a bright stream of blood gushing from her nose and mouth.

Zoe stepped over the teacher and raced to Laya. She looked around the deserted anteroom.

"Let's go! Hurry!"

Laya was frozen, eyes fixed on the growing pool of blood around the teacher's head on the polished floor.

"Laya!"

"She's dead, Mommy."

Zoe crouched beside her daughter. “No, she’s not dead. She’ll be fine, baby.” Inching over, she took the woman’s arm. It twitched and she moaned softly as Zoe took her pulse.

Laya went to Zoe’s side and touched her mother’s long black hair. “I missed you, Mommy.”

“I missed you, too.” A clatter of footsteps from down the hall was getting closer. The teacher was starting to sit up.

Zoe grabbed Laya, stepped outside the building, slammed the door behind them, shutting out the bloodied teacher’s face, her groans, and cries for help.

Across the street, the jogger in the park stood beside his bench, Zoe watched him press a telelink to his lips.

Chapter 36

San Francorp
Medi-Prog Complex

Seka Joraine's stomach was in knots. Dutton had kept her waiting in his reception area for more than thirty miserable minutes. During that time she'd gone over every possible scenario again and again, probed each and every dark alley he might attack from. If she wasn't quick on her feet, with all the right answers on the tip of her tongue, she and Nathan were going down right now.

To calm herself, she studied the photographs that covered the walls, all oversized pictures of San Francorp and Los Anglecorp, with their key Medi-Prog departments—Robotics Surgery, Physical Medicine, Environmental Medicine, Communicable Diseases, Drug Therapy, Organ Health, and Prosthetics. There were also pictures of a large string of Medi-Prog buildings in what used to be known as Arizona and Nevada. They were spread around the sectors, mostly situated in places she'd only vaguely heard of.

But at each facility, in every single picture, Dutton stood at the entrance of the building, smiling widely.

No other people were present in any of the photographs.

Without a doubt, anyone waiting to see the big man in this inner sanctum would instantly get the message that not only Dutton's face, but his fingers were in every aspect of health care for the tri-sector area.

In the short time since Seka left Organ Harvesting, she'd seen that most corporate executive's' offices were not in keeping with the hard times that the general population had to endure. Corporate offices remained spacious and luxurious; they oozed raw power. And they were anything but subtle about it. If size mattered, his massive penthouse office said everything about Dutton's ultimate influence and unshakable power.

As the minutes passed, she became more and more frightened. She needed to pace away her jumpiness, but she forced herself to remain planted in a large contemporary sofa. She would need to appear calm and sincere if she were going to convince the CEO that she was doing what he wanted.

Could she pull it off?

That she'd even allowed herself to become a part of Dutton's plan to spy on Nathan made her realize how desperate she had become. If her self-esteem wasn't top-notch before, it was somewhere in the sewer now. The CEO's undercover scheme was contemptible and unethical.

And she'd not only allowed herself to become a part of it, she'd been eager to have the opportunity.

Somehow, she, Seka Joraine, MD, ordinary individual, had been drawn into the basic struggle between good and evil.

All she'd ever wanted was to be a doctor, to care for people who were sick and needed help. If Organ Harvesting had been the way into the primary medical system, she'd accepted what had to be done. And she'd done it.

But it hadn't worked out.

Organ Harvesting eroded her integrity, made her lose sight of her goals. It brought her down.

Trying to save herself, trying to get away from that kind of medical service, had forced her to become someone else. Someone who could lie, spy, deceitfully use another human being.

Now, she was nothing but a whore, meek and powerless, waiting to be called for a command performance by her pimp.

* * *

"Where was Nathan Quinn last night?" Dutton demanded as she entered his office, not waiting for her to take a seat.

"How would I know? I wasn't supposed to keep track of him twenty-four seven." "That kind of impertinence, Dr. Joraine, is going to put you right back where you came from, if not someplace worse."

"May I sit?" She slid onto a chair before he could answer.

"My assignment was to entice, to determine if Nathan Quinn's a risk."

"And?"

"I enticed him," Seka said. "Quite successfully."

"But is he a risk?"

"That'll take more time."

"Then give me an impression, damn it!"

Seka smiled. "He thinks he's in love with me."

"Not that nonsense, the chemicals did that. What about the fucking risk factor?"

Seka watched Dutton's face turn a dark red. "I told you, that takes longer…I just got started."

"I don't want to hear your excuses. The point is, the man wasn't in his apartment last night. But *you* were there! Explain yourself!"

"Nathan was there when I went to sleep. He was there when I woke up. If he was gone while I was sleeping, I would think your surveillance people would have the answers to those questions."

Dutton stared at her glumly over the tips of his steepled fingers, aware that she was right, although he'd never tell her that. Instead, he said, "There's a possibility Quinn is involved with a fugitive, Dr. Zoe Hidalga."

"She was on the Desisto list of names I gave you, wasn't she?" "Yes."

"He's never mentioned her."

"And you still claim," Dutton said, "you don't know where he went last night?" "If I knew, I would tell you."

He glared at her. "It's really no problem to send you back to Organ Harvesting, Doctor." "I know that."

"Good! So tell me, did anything happen last night that could give us a clue as to where he went?"

Seka offered a hesitant smile. "Sir, Nathan Quinn is a soft, vulnerable man. I truly expected him to spend the night with me in his apartment. I provided him with every possible inducement, chemical and physical. I'm as surprised as you are that he was able to leave me…even for a few minutes, let alone hours."

"But where did he go?" Dutton repeated, his eyes never leaving hers. "There's a thread missing here," he continued, more to himself than to her. He leaned back in his chair. "Did Quinn ever mention a man named Andrew Potter?"

"Chief of Robotics?"

"Yes, him."

"Not a word."

Dutton was silent for a long moment, tapping his fingers on the desk.

"For your sake, Doctor," he finally said, "I hope you're not playing some kind of underhanded game with me." He pointed a pen at her. "That would be a useless exercise in stupidity."

Seka looked at him with a mask of fearful innocence. "I know that, sir."

* * *

When the door closed behind Seka Joraine, Dutton called Commander Potek. "Letting Nathan Quinn out of your sight is inexcusable," he roared over the telelink, not caring whether Potek had his speaker on.

"The CAPO operative was inexperienced," Potek said. "Quinn spotted him and apparently felt threatened." He didn't think it wise to mention the fact that Quinn had slugged the CAPO. "The man has been severely disciplined."

"What good is that now? I need to know where Quinn went." "Why don't we ask him?"

"I'm not ready for a confrontation. There may be others involved. If so, I want them all." "What happened to our spy? I thought she was supposed to be with Quinn again last night."

"I didn't ask for your opinion or your questions. What I want from you are facts. Results!"

Potek was silent.

"Starting immediately," Dutton said, "put twenty-four-hour teams on both Nathan Quinn and Seka Joraine."

* * *

At her desk, Seka rummaged through a pile of documents,

wondering how she could warn Nathan that he was in even more danger than either of them imagined.

In the shortest possible time, she'd gone from being Dutton's hand-picked spy to his sworn enemy, losing a position of advantage to a situation where everything was at risk.

She jumped when the call light on her telelink flashed. Cold sweat coated her back before she realized it was Nathan asking her to meet him for lunch.

"Well?" he prompted, obviously upset.

"Sorry! Lost in what I was doing. Lunch would be fine." "Are you aware—"

"I'll meet you at noon," she interrupted, punching the disconnect button. There could be no taking chances.

She leaned back and stared with mistrust at the telelink.

* * *

When Seka left two hours later to meet Nathan, her computer case file was clear, but she had only the vaguest notion what projects she'd handled, or her solutions for any of them.

They met at the Fast Step restaurant. Nathan could barely wait to speak, jumping right in as soon as they were seated.

"Everything's spinning out of control, Seka. Dutton's coming after me, I know it. I could see it in his eyes today at the department chiefs' meeting."

"We both knew that could happen after last night," Seka said.

"I should have tried to get away from that damn CAPO instead of punching him out. It was an idiotic thing to do."

They grasped each other's hand under the café table.

"But something really horrible has happened," Nathan whispered to Seka. "They've changed X66 to a god dammed VMAS accelerator!"

"What?"

"Dutton announced it to the inner circle this morning. Innovation, he called it, for crissake!"

Seka felt watchful eyes on them. She covered her mouth to hide her reaction. "My God!

What the hell is going on?"

"Right now, all I can think about is Zoe."

"The X66 you gave her, was it the stabilizer or the accelerator?"

"I don't know! It's driving me crazy. I don't dare try to get to Andrew to discuss it, and I don't know how to reach Zoe."

"She's in the Noncorp sector, isn't she?"

"No! I brought her back into the city early this morning."
"You didn't. That's crazy!"

"She's going to steal Laya away from the boarding school. Don't ask me how. I couldn't get any of it out of her."

"Doesn't she realize the CAPOs will be watching the school, that she'll almost certainly be caught?"

"There was no stopping her, Seka. Besides, she may be CAPO-listed but she's a low priority Desisto candidate. And if she makes it, we're to meet this evening at a safe house."

"Nathan! She shouldn't have come back; she's put us all in danger." She told him about her meeting with Dutton. "What do we do if she's been given the accelerator?"

"I don't know. There's so much I don't know about it. The effective absorption rate is critical, and if there's time, I need to get my hands on uncontaminated X66."

Seka pressed a knee against his leg. "Be careful, Nathan. They're already suspicious. If they catch you at *anything*, Dutton will have the CAPOs pick you up…you'll be finished."

"Our only chance is to get out of the city as soon as possible. All of us!"

"Dutton must be having both of us watched," Seka said. "We don't dare leave until after dark."

"I feel so god dammed useless. Don't know enough to be in the middle of this kind of mess."

She clutched Nathan's thigh. "Maybe not, but that's where we are. Right smack in the middle."

Chapter 37

San Francorp

"Laya! We have to hurry. Let's go!"

But her daughter stood dazed, wide-eyed, unfocused. She refused to move.

Zoe yanked her away from the school entrance, pulled her in the direction of the underground electro-magno station. If they could just catch a pod and vanish before the CAPOs get to them, they might have a chance.

But Laya remained rigid; Zoe had to drag her.

"Laya, we have to go. If we're ever going to be together, we have to move now."

The jogger started to run toward them. Zoe forced herself to turn away and keep moving.

"Mommy, I'm scared."

Zoe couldn't stop herself, she had to look back. The man was running faster toward them.

"He's trying to catch us," Laya said, following her mother's stare. "Is it because you hurt Ms. Harper?"

"I had to get you out of there, Laya. There was no other way." "But—"

Words spilled out of Zoe's mouth. "I didn't want to hurt her, but it was our only chance of having a life together. You have to trust me, Laya."

Zoe kept tugging at Laya's arm.

"Do you remember 'Skip-to-my-Lou'?" Fear twisted her gut into knots. Laya nodded.

"Let's see how many verses we can sing between here and the underground."

Far-off sirens filled the air, the distinctive wail of CAPO vehicles warned that they had a very short head start. Zoe began to skip, taking large steps, pulling Laya along. Her breath came in loud gasps; her heart tore at her chest. Finally, Laya moved into Zoe's rhythm. They skipped faster and faster, mouthed the ancient children's song.

Skip, skip, skip to my Lou, Skip, skip, skip to my Lou, Skip, skip, skip to my Lou, Skip to my Lou, my darlin'.

Zoe's legs grew heavier and heavier; she had to fight to keep up the pace, to keep from falling. The sirens drew closer, louder.

"Three, mommy!" Laya said as they finally entered the underground electro-magno escalator. "We sang three verses!"

Zoe looked behind them. The jogger was close, lumbering along while trying to work with his communicator. He may have been dressed in sports gear, but he wasn't an athlete. He could barely keep going.

"One more verse, Laya," she stuttered, struggling to breathe. She tore through her pockets for Nathan's travel card.

Where the hell did I put it?

Without the card, they would be stopped at the electronic force field.

The sirens screeched above them now. Zoe and Laya ran the rest of the way down the escalator just as an express pod pulled up to the passenger platform.

"Another verse, Mommy?"

"Okay," she wheezed. The loud whoop of a CAPO pursuit vehicle hiccupped above them: Loud, demanding, penetrating.

The jogger jumped off the escalator and screamed as the pod's yellow boarding light flashed departure. "Halt! Don't…board that … pod!"

"Run, Laya! Run!" Zoe tore at her pockets. "… card … dammit …"

Laya stumbled at the gateway. Zoe yanked her up, kept running, fumbling through her pockets until she found the plastin travel card in her breast pocket. She slammed it through the slot and they bolted through the gate.

The runner came to a grinding halt as he smashed into the reenergized force field.

The pod's light flicked from yellow to red as Zoe and Laya jumped through the closing doors, crumpled onto the floor. Laya looked up and pointed toward the man.

"We beat him, Mommy!"

* * *

They transferred from line to line within the meandering transportation system until Zoe was certain no one was following them. At first, she was suspicious of every person who entered the pod. But after several transfers she was convinced that, at least for now, they had gotten away from the CAPOs.

She tried to keep their movements as inconspicuous as possible, but they still attracted the attention of other riders. Many of the pod's passengers openly stared at the mother-daughter combo. Zoe knew she stood out in her fake Corporit clothes, and Laya should have been in school at this time of day.

"You look sick, Mommy," Laya said, interrupting a question about her schoolwork.

"Just tired, Laya." She thrust her hands into her pockets to hide their tremors.

"But you're getting so skinny."

"I know. I haven't been eating the way I should without you around to take care of me.

And it's no fun cooking just for me."

"We're going to be together all the time now, aren't we?" She snuggled closer and wrapped her arms around Zoe's waist.

"And we're going to a beautiful place where there are real trees and flowers and animals," Zoe said softly. "You'll love it."

"You mean like the zoo?"

Zoe laughed. "No, not like the zoo. Those aren't real animals anymore. This is a place where we can live…and you can see living birds in the trees."

"Really?"

"Wait and see."

Laya bounced up and down on the seat. "Tell me! Tell me about it!"

Zoe placed a finger to her lips, bent down, pressed her

forehead against Laya's, and whispered. "A long time ago, the earth was very much like this place we're going to. Wherever you looked you could see trees and plants and animals and birds."

"What happened?"

"They disappeared. People didn't understand how important they were." Laya's eyes widened.

"No one cared?"

"Some people did. They cared very much. But no one listened to them until it was too late."

"But, Mommy, you said we're going where they still have all of those things."

Zoe curled her fingers into a globe-like shape. "Yes. They're in a big, magical place that covers the land as far as you can see; some of these places are as tall as the largest buildings in San Francorp."

"And that's where we're going, where you and me are going to live together there?"

"From now on."

Laya was silent for a moment. "Why was that man chasing us?"

Zoe kissed the top of Laya's head. "There are people who think we shouldn't be together. But you're my little girl, and *nothing* is going to separate us again."

* * *

They arrived at Andrew Potter's safe house late that afternoon; Zoe punched in the security number and the door unlocked. Laya ran to a large chair and bounced up and down.

"Look, Mommy! Isn't this fun?"

Zoe collapsed on the sofa and passed out. When she awoke with a start, Laya was running her fingers through her hair, a worried look on her face.

"What happened to you, Mommy?"

"Too much running, I think." She felt as though her life was draining away with every breath. She blinked several times but her vision was clouded and darkness kept closing in. She forced herself to smile at Laya, who seemed very far away.

"Isn't this a nice place? It belongs to an old friend."

Zoe wanted to do something for her daughter. Perform some simple task. Maybe fix her something to eat, provide an act of love or kindness that her little girl would always remember. But every time she tried to get up, something crushed down on her chest and pinned her to the sofa.

"See if there's anything in the refrigerator for you to eat."

Zoe watched the blurry outline of Laya move to the small kitchen, open the refrigerator, and look inside.

"There's milk and cheese. I'll just pour some milk for us."

"Not for me, sweetheart. I need to rest."

Zoe wanted to close her eyes and never open them again. Her body seemed to sink down, then farther down, until it was as though she'd enmeshed into the fibers of the sofa.

"You go ahead and eat, Laya." Her words seemed so far away; she was in a deep cavern, calling out to her daughter.

"How long do we have to stay here, Mommy?"

"Not very long," Zoe said. Her eyes closed even though she fought to keep them open. Her voice came in waves, sounded strange. Loud, like a bellowing beast. She swallowed hard, fought against a flood of rising bile that blasted her throat.

Zoe heard Laya set the milk and cheese on a table next to her. "Tell me about the animals and flowers again," she said. Then without warning, she burst into tears.

"What's wrong?" Zoe said, her eyes now open, yet everything around her was turning black.

"I don't deserve to go there with you."

Zoe listened to the sound of her daughter's voice and reached out until she could caress her cheek. "Why would you say such a thing? No one deserves it more than you."

"It's my fault Daddy died."

"No, Laya! It wasn't your fault." Zoe opened her arms and Laya moved into her embrace. "Your daddy died because he was very, very sick with a bad disease. That's why he died."

"But they took me away. I *must* have done something

wrong, Mommy."

She tried to squeeze Laya close to her, but a draining numbness had settled into her arms. "No, no! You didn't do anything wrong. It was me. I was so upset after Daddy died, they didn't think I could take care of you."

"I'm not much trouble, Mommy. I could have helped."

"I tried to tell them that, but they wouldn't listen."

"Then you're not angry with me?" Laya asked, her tears falling onto her mother's cheek.

"I wasn't ever angry with you. Not once. I love you."

Laya threw her arms around Zoe's neck. "I love you, too, Mommy."

Chapter 38

Medi-Prog
Nathan Quinn's Office

Bright red letters blinked on Nathan Quinn's computer screen.

A news alert scrolled across the monitor with the latest Corporit headlines.

VMAS VACCINE READY FOR PUBLIC INOCULATION ... VMAS STABILIZER WILL SAVE LIVES OF INFECTED POPULATION ... MEDICAL UPDATES TO FOLLOW

A world filled with lies...lies about Corporit care...lies about the stabilizer. Lies.

He reached into his pocket and pulled out his telelink. The numerical keys blurred. He was stymied. How could he help Zoe survive?

What could he do? Where could he go? Who could he call?

Dutton and his system have me exactly where he wants me—hog-tied and helpless.

Nathan sat on the edge of his desk chair. He was jumpy and couldn't stop his hands from shaking. Right now, CAPOs were following, listening, monitoring every single one in his messages. No matter who he reached out to, Emory Dutton or one of his hired thugs would be there waiting to dissect every word, evaluate every gesture.

Nathan's heart thumped painfully and he had a sudden stabbing headache.

When he focused on the chain of events, he knew just from the timing of Zoe receiving the stabilizer that she was given the killer accelerator.

She would die very soon without intervention.

He had to make the right connection…now! He had to find the right person to get the real stabilizer, or it was all over for her.

He looked out through the wall of glass and stared at Seka's empty desk.

Nathan needed her to be here, needed to have a sense that there was some kind of future for the two of them. That there was something worth living for.

But he'd sent her to the safe house to make sure Zoe made it, was even alive. If the worst happened and Zoe died, Seka was to take Laya away, if she was there, and hide her. No matter what, they would try to save Zoe's daughter.

His skin felt swollen, tight; he gnawed at a thumbnail. He had to come up with something, some plan that would put the effective, medically safe X66 compound in his hands.

One thing was certain. There would be no help from Andrew Potter. He'd made that clear. He was out of the picture for now. If he were caught aiding a fugitive, it would jeopardize the whole Defy network. Dutton was already suspicious about the Robotic Surgery chief. At the moment, it was all supposition…smoke and mirrors, as Andrew said. The CEO had no real proof against him…yet. But Dutton was inventive and if he could prove *anything,* Andrew would be eliminated.

Yes, the robotic genius is definitely out of the picture.

In only three days, Andrew's covert life had broadsided Nathan. Before then, he'd never really examined or appreciated all the automatic privileges that were the foundations of his life. He'd had it easy. Taken his family perks, everything else for granted.

He knew that without his family's connections, he would have been nothing but a drone, subject to the will of the corporations and its micromanagement of society. Like Zoe. Like Seka.

Was that how Dutton viewed Seka, a mechanical drone he could turn on and off whenever he damned well pleased?

No doubt.

And Nathan? Either do what he was told or lose the security of the Corporit tit.

The hell with it. Push all the buttons you want, Emory Dutton. Seka and I have disconnected.

He slid back into his chair, drummed his fingers on the desktop. No matter which mental doorway he went through, all he found was an empty room. No windows, no doors.

No exit.

* * *

Nathan went to his parents' apartment, stationed himself at the kitchen table, and tried to wait patiently for his father's return. After several minutes, he grew restless and moved into the living room to think about what he would to say to him. He hated having to ask for his father's help. He hadn't done that in a long time. But Zoe's life was on the line and he could not allow his pride to interfere with saving her.

The truth was, he wished he'd never known or gotten word about the availability of the Chief of DP position.

When he'd heard of the job opening, he deliberately did not tell his family of his decision to try for the position. After he'd nailed it, it was still difficult for him to explain why—his parents lived and breathed their work, saving lives. Desisto's sole mission was to take lives.

His father never really understood that Nathan was a basic, uncomplicated person. It even took Nathan a long time to learn it about himself, to understand that although he was motivated by idealism when he went into medicine, the system had disillusioned him. His parents never could accept that now all he wanted was a job that would provide him with security. Nothing more.

For him, books and music became his passions. Medicine had been nothing but a huge mistake.

When he signed on as Chief of DP, and finally told his parents, they congratulated him, and that was that. Their reaction surprised Nathan. He thought they would want a blow-by-blow break-down of what the job entailed. But that never happened.

Now he wished they'd had that discussion.

Nathan realized how naïve he was. He was in way over his head.

* * *

When his father finally came home, Nathan could see he was surprised to see him, but it was obvious he was also pleased.

"How's the new job going?" his father asked after they embraced.

Nathan ignored the question for the moment. They sat down together on the plush sofa, but he still hesitated. He looked around at the many paintings in the room, mostly of different species of trees and forests. The canvasses were not only vibrant, but heavily textured in a way that drew the viewer right into the wooded landscapes. His father had chosen these particular paintings. The pictures of nude women staring out of windows, or into empty space, were certainly his mother's choices.

My mother, the dreamer.

Nathan turned to scrutinize his father; something he hadn't done in a long time.

He was a big man; the sofa barely contained his tall, stocky body. Since he'd retired, the beginnings of a spare tire had settled around his middle, and his shoulders had begun to slump. It made Nathan sad; his dad was growing old. Still, when he looked into his eyes, he saw a man of passion, someone who cared, wanted to cure the world of every disease. Corporit, Noncorp, and Aught. It didn't matter to him. People were people and he didn't like to see anyone suffer.

"You haven't answered my question," his father said.

"It's complicated. I'm not sure this Medi-Prog placement was the right move for me." He tried to change the subject. "Where's Mom?"

His father's face lost its color. "You know where she is. At the hospital making rounds. The sixty-retirement axe hasn't hit her yet." His father turned away, but not before Nathan saw his lips pull into a tight, straight line. "Since I *moved on*, as they say, I think I bore the hell out of her."

"That's unfair, Dad. I mean, you seem to spend almost as much time at the hospital as you used to. I'm lucky to catch you at home."

"It's really no one's fault," his father said, continuing as though Nathan hadn't spoken. "After you left home, our interests mostly centered on our individual medical involvements." He looked into Nathan's eyes, then turned away and gazed across the room. "I don't think she cares much what I do anymore; I feel like I've lost her respect."

"That's not true. I don't believe it. Maybe you're being oversensitive."

"Hey, it's a big comedown. No one knows that better than me. I used to be the CNC Physician-in-Charge. Now I'm an armchair consultant. It's quite a nosedive. I'm the first to admit my world has narrowed considerably."

"But you're as involved and busy as ever, aren't you?"

His father managed a dry cough that Nathan knew was supposed to pass for a laugh. "Communicable diseases take on a whole new perspective when you're talking about low-level stuff like a mundane study of strep mutation. Boring…boring…boring! I'd much rather be researching VMAS and intercepting its viral-induced coma. Now that's valuable." He smiled, but the humor avoided his eyes. "I just miss the action…being at the center of things."

Nathan remained silent.

"Wait a minute! Did you say you think Desisto wasn't the right move for you?"

Nathan shrugged noncommittally.

"You didn't get much help from me, but I know you called in a lot of your own favors to snatch up that so called prize." A deep frown mapped his father's forehead. "You've barely gotten your head into it. Don't tell me you're looking for a way out already?"

"Have you ever worked for Emory Dutton?"

"No, thank you!" His father gave him a dismissive wave of the hand. "So the man's a bastard and doesn't give a damn about people. He didn't get to the top of the heap by being Mr. Nice Guy."

Nathan said nothing for a long moment. "You don't really mean that, do you, Dad? We both know he's an immoral son-of-a-bitch. I wish you'd tried to talk me out of settling into that prize post."

"Nathan, I just couldn't understand why Dutton ever gave you the position in the first place. Your family name alone should have kept you out of the running from the start. If you would've told me what you were doing, it might have saved you from being involved in something that's beneath you. There's so much bad blood between Dutton and our family."

His father tapped his knee. "There's only one reason he would allow you into his enterprise—to find a way to use you, to get to your mother and me. Trust me, he'll do everything he can to discredit our family name. That's the kind of despicable man he is."

"Yes, he's a devious son-of-a-bitch."

"No doubt, yet under his leadership they've come up with not only a VMAS stabilizer, but a vaccine as well. I suppose you have to give the devil his due. And as much as I hate to say it, I call that a job well done. I envy the accomplishment."

"You don't know the whole truth, Dad?"

"Know what?"

Nathan wanted to delay telling his father what was really happening, but he didn't want to lose this unexpected moment of shared intimacy. Nathan pointed past his father to a picture on the piano.

"Remember that day, Dad?"

It was a photograph of the two of them on their last camping trip in the woods at Lake Tahoe—just before all wooded areas were declared out of bounds. Groves of dying, falling limbs and whole trees forest areas too dangerous to enter.

I was only eight. Can't believe thirty years have gone by.

The photo showed his dad with a shit-eating grin on his face and Nathan hugging him around the middle. They both looked very happy.

"That was a great weekend, Dad."

His father gave him a wide smile—the same kind of smile that transformed him into the person in the photograph.

Could he really trust this man? A man who walked around the dinner table proselytizing about medicine to him and his mother? Who was always quick to point out that his son never got anything quite right? A man he loved, but who made him feel like he could never measure up?

It has to be you, Dad, or Zoe dies.

"I need you, Dad. I need your help to save a friend's life. And, Dad, I can't minimize how dangerous this could be for you and Mom if you decide to help. But either you help me, or she dies."

The silence crept into every corner of the room while his father picked at a loose thread on the arm of the sofa. Finally, he mumbled, "Still the same kid…always trying to fix things, whether it's a person or a broken bicycle."

Nathan smiled. "Sometimes, I wish I was that kind of person again. Somewhere along the way, I lost that inner fire."

"Son, you wouldn't be here if you had."

Nathan squeezed his father's arm. "I must have picked that up from someone I know." The corners of his father's mouth turned up again. "Maybe so, son."

Nathan took a long, deep breath. "Dad, starting tomorrow, everyone with VMAS is getting a contaminated X66—designer-engineered to kill them. And as far as I can tell, only Corporit CEOs and their executive staff will be excluded…they'll be the only recipients of an actual stabilizer."

His father's eyes widened. "Are you sure? You're talking about the new VMAS stabilizer?"

"Dutton plans to not only rid the population of VMAS; he wants to reduce the population to a more *manageable* number. That's what Desisto Processing is all about. Dutton claims it's because of our declining resources, but who the hell knows what the truth is or what his real agenda is?"

His dad stood abruptly, his face a bright red. "Not even Dutton would do that! " He reached a trembling hand out to his son, drew him out of the sofa. "…would he?"

"I think my friend Zoe Hidalga has probably already been given the contaminated accelerant." Nathan took his father's hand, looked into his tear filled eyes.

He folded Nathan into an embrace, whispered in his ear. "Are you sure, son?"

"Yes, Dad, I am."

His father hugged him tighter and a wave of tremors shook his body as he sobbed. "Nathan, what have we become?"

Chapter 39

HospitalCorp
Infectious Diseases

Dr. Tris Quinn entered the fourth floor corridor as though he were still an attending MD, an integral part of the everyday Corporit hospital system instead of a forced retiree housed in the laboratory. He probably should have been grateful to be still involved with the research and consulting staff at all. But he didn't feel either grateful or lucky.

At the huge central telemetry island, he studied the incoming computer graphics of the different patients' hearts and biorhythms. His body relaxed and he was mesmerized by the minute-to-minute displays of blood work, radiology, binary information, all on each individual as it scrolled across the multiple screens. For the first time in two years, he felt like someone at the top of his game again, someone with a real purpose.

This is where I belong.

Had it only been thirty-five years since his medical initiation? It seemed longer, and although he confessed it to no one, not even his wife, he felt older than sixty-two.

It had been so different in the beginning, before Corporit took over governing the medical world. It had certainly been a fallible system, but at least the majority of people were cared for in a humane and honest way.

He had to slow himself down. He was only here to be help his son's friend, yet a growing anger clouded his thinking. He wanted to reach out and smash the entities that had turned caregivers into murderers … Corporit stars like Emory Dutton, who cared nothing about people.

What a fool! I gave up the fight, the ideals, so I could stay relevant. In the end, I went along with everything. Toed the line and stopped asking questions. And one day, I awoke to a world of medical management that I no longer recognized or approved of.

Nathan was right—he was taking a big chance But wasn't it about time to step up, time to do *something?*

He still had a current Ident-card because of his consult activity—it could help him pull this off, help him slide through this dangerous situation.

Damn well better do it right, or Nathan and Rebecca will go down with me.

"Dr. Quinn! What a pleasure," a young intern said. "Haven't run into you for a while. Where have you been hiding?"

Tris nodded and smiled.

Last thing I need right now is recognition by a lot of people.

"Hey, Tomas, have you decided to stick with infectious diseases? I thought internal medicine was going to be your thing. " Tris turned back to the screens, making it apparent this wasn't a good time to reconnect.

Tomas said, "We can talk another time, sir. Maybe I'll see you in Corpmall later."

Tris let his breath out slowly as the intern walked away. Before he could figure out exactly what to do next, Rebecca startled him by grabbing his arm. Her blue eyes looked puzzled. But she pressed against him and whispered, "And what are you doing here, Dr. Quinn? You weren't scheduled for a consult today."

"Dr. Rebecca Quinn. How good to see you." Seeing his wife made him feel safer, surer "Just taking care of a few things."

"Tris, you're only making it more difficult to give up this whole business."

He gave her a look that would tell her something important had happened. He asked, "Are you on the way home now?"

"In about half an hour," Rebecca said. She never took her eyes away from his. There were many serious questions written in her body language.

He smiled as though he didn't have a care, but his heart felt like it had permanently lodged in his throat.

"I'll meet you downstairs. Wait for me." He leaned over and kissed her cheek. When he was sure she was off the ward, he sat down in one of the monitoring chairs that surrounded the island and casually looked around, surveyed everything.

The corridors looked sterile—no paintings, walls an icy white. Why had he never noticed that before? But hospital décor had never held his interest; it was always more important to come in and get to work.

For the first time that he could remember, he really paid attention to his environment. It was pretty damn stark, and this particular floor was for the corporate elite. He didn't even want to compare it to the average worker-bee accommodations, with their get-well-quick-or-die ambiance.

Some deep breaths slowed his racing heart. He jacked into one of the computer boards, tapped into the information on a patient he'd been called in to provide a second opinion about recently. Then he randomly scrolled through the long list of VMAS patients until he came to a Lolo Lang.

Her history told the story: Vice President of Infocorp, a PR corporation, for more than thirty years.

Public Information, my ass. Infocorp's more like the biggest, most successful propaganda machine in the Corporit system.

Lolo had contracted VMAS right after the "sixty" axe took effect.

He scrolled through her records until he came to the Advance Directive. In no uncertain terms, it stated she wanted no medications or heroic machinations to save her life, especially if she contracted a fatal illness.

Who was the case doctor?

None. Her end-of-life instructions had guaranteed that paradigm. All she had now to look after her was a case manager.

Yeah, she and fifty others with the same overworked nurse

tech.

Without further investigation, Quinn punched in a X66 stabilizing compound order and sent it to the unit pharmacy. The directions stated that the patch was to be applied to her arm immediately. A short consulting note stated the patient had changed her Advance Directive.

Her executive rank guaranteed compliance and he knew the patch would be a life- sustaining stabilizer, rather than the VMAS accelerator patch.

They won't pick up on this for a long time, if ever. And Lolo Lang will probably be dead by then. Just as she directed.

He was uneasy, though. He needed to see the woman to be sure he wasn't harming her in any way.

* * *

Tris Quinn stood outside Lolo Lang's room, not knowing what to expect, or how he could backtrack if things didn't go as expected.

Entering the darkened space, he noticed immediately that she was in the coma-ridden stages of VMAS; her breathing was slow and difficult. This kind of horrible death rattle predicted that the end would come shortly. No life-sustaining paraphernalia attached, as she had requested, but at this point, nothing could ever change her outcome. VMAS *would* take her life.

He started to turn away but his gaze caught a burgundy repli-rose in an antique cut glass vase. He bent over and read the note sitting next to it.

I love you, Mom.

He sat down in the small chair next to the bed and listened to the painful breathing of Lolo Lang, a human being in transition from this life to whatever the universe had to offer.

"Although you don't know it, Lolo, today, you saved a life." He reached for her frail, lifeless hand and as he moved to leave, her fingers pressed his.

* * *

Tris walked down the hall to the unit pharmacy to pick up

the X66 he'd ordered under Lolo Lang's name.

If I don't pull this off, this really could be my very last day in Infectious Disease—in medicine. But I'm going to pick up that damn stabilizer and sign off on it with my sloppy handwriting. And just maybe for once in my life, my messy scroll will turn out to be a good thing.

He glanced at his watch and his step picked up. Rebecca would be downstairs waiting. He knew his wife, his Becky. She would have done exactly the same thing, if Nathan had asked her.

He had a smile on his face.

CHAPTER 40

San Francorp
Defy Safe House

Searing light stretched across the horizon like a flaming backdrop to the attacking, flesh- eating Aughts. They spewed from mountains of steaming garbage like hungry, blood-sucking creatures, scavenging for food across the black, lifeless debris. The screaming gargoyle faces grew closer and closer, and the acrid smell of their rotting bodies smothered the air.

They surrounded Storm. They surround Zoe.

Godan stepped out from the clot of Aughts. He yanked at a long, leather leash; gave a vicious tug and pulled Laya up from the hungry masses.

Zoe could hear her own voice in the terrorizing dream. *"Layaaaaa!"*

Godan reeled the struggling girl toward him.

"Mommy! Help me!"

Zoe struggled to get to her. She turned to plead with Storm to help save her daughter. But he had vanished. She was alone. And her daughter's screams continued to echo in her head.

Godan's laughter tore through the air. He yanked at Laya's arm, raised it high, and smashed it down across his knee; a loud, sickening snap echoed from everywhere.

Zoe bolted upright.

She blinked to clear away the threatening shadows that jumped out all around her.

Someone was unlocking the front door.

She uncurled herself from her sleeping daughter, grabbed a metal sculpture, and stumbled across the living room. Before she could reach the entry, the darkness exploded in a flood of bright light from the building hallway. A startled woman held up her arms for protection.

"Zoe! Don't! I'm Seka Joraine … Nathan sent me."

"Who?" Zoe let go of the sculpture. It thumped onto the floor and rolled away.

"Mommy, what's wrong?"

Zoe looked from Seka to her daughter. She couldn't focus on either of them; they were only smeary blurs of movement. She was soaked in icy perspiration, her head throbbed with pain, and flashes of lightning seared her eyes.

"Zoe?"

Who is she calling? Is that my name?

Disconnected sounds rattled, echoed in her head. She reached for Laya, but she was so far away. Zoe fell to her knees and collapsed in a heap.

Nathan's friend was next to her, checking her pulse. She could still hear her daughter calling her. The two voices fused into a jumble of bouncing sounds.

"Zoe!" Seka shouted. She shook Zoe's shoulders. "Where's the patch?"

"Leave my mommy alone!"

"Your mommy's sick. We have to help her."

Zoe moaned, twisted back and forth.

"Help me get her to the sofa," Seka said.

Zoe could hear their voices; feel their hands on her body as she swam through a dark, gooey nothingness. She tried to waken herself, but before she could surface, more pain cramped her muscles, dragged her down again.

"Mommy!" Laya cried, shaking her arm.

From far away, she watched the woman grab a floor lamp and tilt it over her. "Laya, hold this!"

Zoe watched them through the wrong end of a telescope; they were like wavering dots far, far away. Fingers moved across her arms and legs, up and down her body.

"Stop it!" Zoe shouted. "You're hurting me." Her muscles cramped tighter as the hands searched her body, sending every part of her into violent spasms. She punched out at empty air. The lamp crashed away. She fought them and sat up gasping for air. Bile burned her throat, then gushed from her mouth.

"Damn it, Zoe! I can stop the pain. Where did you put the patch? The VMAS stabilizer? It has to come off. Do you hear me?"

"Leave her alone!" Laya screamed again.

Seka moved in very close. Zoe stared at the woman with unfocused eyes. She pounded her fists into her gut, over and over.

"Nathan…gave it to me."

"They fooled him…it's no good…do you understand?"

"No good?"

"That's right, Zoe…no good! Where is it?"

Her eyes closed, her head dropped. The desperate voice faded. Zoe was falling through space. It was a long way down, but she knew when she landed, sleep would take away all the pain. She would finally find peace. Her heart fluttered like a drum out of sync.

"ZOEEEE! WAAKE UP! VEEMAAS PAATCCH!"

Someone was there with her in the darkness. Someone was reaching out to her.

"Elliot? Elliot! Is that you? I'm here!"

She wanted to touch him. She stretched out, tried to touch his face, half-hidden in the deep shadows; it disintegrated and like shredded paper, it flew away. But it wasn't Elliot. It was—

"WAAKE UP, ZOEEE!"

Storm!

Zoe looked deep into his soft, comforting, amber eyes. He was trying to tell her something. A golden light unfolded, curled out from within Storm, and rode a misty fog. It radiated out until it encircled her. She was surrounded in healing warmth that held her, embraced her, stopped her from falling into nothingness. For long moments, she hung suspended, then her arms lifted and she reached up to Storm so he could pull her from the darkness.

"Where is it, Zoe? Where's the stabilizer?"

Laya bent over her, tears flooded her face. "Tell her, Mommy! Please!"

Zoe raised a hand and pointed. “My right shoulder.”

“I’ve looked there,” Seka said, her voice tense.

“Can’t see it. Have to scratch it off.”

Seka’s nails raked hard against Zoe’s skin.

Chapter 41

Corporit Zone
Safe House

Nathan unlocked the safe house door and frantically flipped off the light, plunging the room into sudden darkness. His heart raced and he was disoriented; a rush of adrenalin made him want to run. He stumbled, jammed a knee into a chair, and forced himself to stop. Just stop.

He took in deep breaths, inched forward trying to adjust to the inky blackness around him. He whispered, "Seka? Are you here?"

"I'm here." Her arms encircled him and he felt her rapid breath course through him until after a few moments they were inhaling and exhaling as one.

He moved away, hands in front of him to detect any obstacles, stepped toward the street light seeping through the window blinds. Seka held onto his jacket, followed in his steps.

He said over his shoulder, "Sorry I'm so late. I came as soon as I could. Dutton's people are everywhere. They're not even trying to hide anymore. It's as if they're daring me to slip up, do something really stupid so they can run me in." He poked a finger through the closed blinds, looked up and down the street.

"We knew it would be like this," Seka said.

"I dodged in and out of office buildings, zigzagged through different malls until I lost them. At least I think I lost them. Damn, it's like there's a big cat out there toying with us."

Seka pressed hard against his back, her arms squeezed him up against her. "It doesn't make any difference," she said, her voice cutting through the darkness in a breathless whisper. "As long as you're here, as long as you're here with me."

He spun around and gathered her into his arms. She trembled against him and the wetness of the tears rolled down her cheeks onto his face. "I'm sorry I worried you."

"All that matters is that you're here now," she said. "That's all I care about. I kept thinking of how I couldn't bear the thought of you out there alone, of never seeing you again. I still keep thinking the same thing, saying the same words over and over." She laid her head on his chest.

"How's Zoe?" Nathan said.

"She's asleep. But we almost lost her. It was very close."

"And her daughter?"

"Also asleep. Exhausted."

Nathan sighed. "I was afraid to ask. I never really believed she'd get Laya away from that school. How in hell did she pull it off?"

"When I got here she was in no condition to tell me anything." Seka laughed softly. "But she sure as hell was strong enough to try and kill me when I came into the apartment."

"Are you kidding?"

"If you think anyone is going to threaten that mama and her cub, think again. Even half- dead, she was ready to fight." Seka slipped out of his arms. "Did you get the stabilizer?"

Nathan smiled. "Yes."

"We'd better get it to her. I scraped off the original one, the accelerator."

"I'll go with you."

He took the package from his pocket. Once in the bedroom, Seka closed the blinds and pulled the drapes before turning on the bedside lamp.

Mother and daughter lay curled in each other's arms. "She's been through a lot," Nathan said.

Zoe's breathing was slow and even; she didn't even stir as Seka applied the patch to her arm.

"The last thing I wanted to do was draw my family into this whole mess," Nathan whispered. "But in the end, my father was the only one I could turn to. Without him, I never would have found an unadulterated lot of X66 in time."

"It must have been difficult for you to have to ask."

"It was. But it became one of those rare moments when

Dad and I were on the same page. The man stepped right up. There was no stopping him. I couldn't have if I'd tried." He smiled widely. "I'm pretty proud of him…and of myself, I guess."

Nathan finished examining Zoe, then placed a hand lightly on her forehead. "Her color looks good, don't you think?"

Seka nodded. "The tremors are gone, too. We'll know more when she wakes up."

They tiptoed back into the living room, turned the light on again. Nathan sat down and pulled Seka onto his lap.

"How did your dad get the stabilizer?"

"He wouldn't tell me. Said there were some things I didn't need to know. But it was weird; he looked really satisfied and it's the happiest I've seen my mom in a long time." He looked at Seka. "My parents would adore you, think you're wonderful, the way I do. I wish you could meet them."

"Maybe I will one day."

He studied Seka's face. Worry was etched on her forehead and her lips were pressed into a tight straight line. He kissed her and her mouth softened under his.

"Have I told you lately how much I love you?" he said.

"I never get tired of hearing it."

"And I have this sinking feeling that none of this is real. That you're not really here with me." He tightened his arms around her, his lips slid to her neck. "Are you really all right?"

"I'm really scared."

"Me, too. I'm used to a much more predictable lifestyle. I don't know how Andrew Potter does it, how he can live undercover, keep people like Dutton away, and hold down a complicated job. It's beyond me. I haven't even figured out how we're all going to get out of this mess. The only thing I do know, is we have to get away tonight. Daylight will be our worst enemy."

"Where will we go, where will we live?" Seka said, her face drawn and worried.

Nathan remained silent. He held onto her, afraid she would

slip away if she knew the truth. He had no idea how they were going to survive. All of this was a wild leap of faith.

"We're leaving and we're not coming back, is that it?" she said. "I mean, you really mean it?"

"Do you want to live like this?"

"No, I don't want to ever come back. Not ever."

"Leave now, while you can get away!" Zoe said, startling them. She stood in the doorway, swaying back and forth. "Laya and I can make it back to the domes on our own."

"You shouldn't be up." Seka slid off Nathan's lap, started toward her. "You need to rest for as long as you can. Besides, we're not going anywhere without you."

"You've already saved my life. I can't ask you to keep risking your own."

"We can't stay," Nathan said, "and neither can you. You're not only DP listed, they'll probably have you nailed with criminal charges for taking Laya. The CAPOs can legally shoot you on sight."

"We're leaving the Corporits for the same reasons you are," Seka said. "They'll hunt us down, trap us, kill us, too. Besides, we can't be a part of this anymore…when they start giving the accelerant—"

"Accelerant?"

"If Seka hadn't removed the patch you were wearing, you'd be in a coma, or dead, by now," Nathan said. "They've turned X66 into a delivery system for extermination."

Zoe's hand shot up to her throat. When she spoke, her voice was barely audible. "A VMAS accelerant?"

"They're telling VMAS patients they're getting a stabilizer, but in reality, anyone with VMAS will be terminated. Corporit, Noncorp, or Aught," Nathan said. "Only CEOs and their executive staffs who are infected with the disease will get the real stabilizer."

"And they'll find every infected person on the grid," Seka said. "Either through the CARE units or via Corporit medical records."

"Exactly!" Nathan said. "They'll dispense the bogus medication and the population will be sanitized within three days."

"All those people!" Zoe said. "They can't get away with that."

"Yes, they can," Seka said. "A new VMAS vaccine will be the carrot than reels them all in."

"A vaccine? But that's wonderful!"

"It should be, but after they trumpet the breakthrough, they'll also bring in everyone with VMAS for the purge."

"Every individual will get either the accelerant or the vaccine, depending on whether they already have VMAS," Seka said, sitting back down on the sofa. "Only they won't be told that."

"Lots of fanfare, speeches, publicity," Nathan said. "The purge will be over in no more than three days."

"Efficient!" Red spots of anger spotted Zoe's pale cheeks. "You have to give them that."

"Dutton's master plan. The man is always one step ahead of everyone."

"At least we've now given you the *real* stabilizer," Seka said "You're not going to die."

Zoe walked across the room and sat down on the sofa between the two of them. "You're telling me the truth, not some fairy tale to make me feel better?"

"I could never lie to you, Zoe," Nathan said. "You should know that." Seka nodded in agreement.

Zoe smiled at them, ran her hand down Nathan's arm. "How can I ever thank you enough, old camp buddy?"

He kissed her on both cheeks. "I'd do it again."

Chapter 42

Noncorps Sector
The Caplac Domes

Asher Wind Storm's mind swirled in an eddy of troubling thoughts. No matter how much he willed it, each abstraction, each fragment of an idea refused to melt away into the night's mysterious ether; it all clung to him like the finest particles of dust.

He gazed into the embers of a small fire as though all answers could be drawn from the flash of leaping flames.

Zoe's and Laya's plight…the death of his dear friend, Arina, they all invaded his thoughts, clouded his mind, fragmented his focus.

Zoe Hidalga.

He knew she stood in a whirling vortex of transition between life and death. A space where life-altering decisions require an independent focus, the kind of concentration of purpose and strength that must take root in her heart if she is to survive.

His thoughts continued to drift, drift; riding, rising along tendrils of smoke that soared toward the upper reaches of this oldest dome. Outside there was vast abandoned land that stretched to the enclosed and dying city of San Francorp. But here in the far reaches of the new Noncorp community was a richness of life, a microcosm of primal Earth that once swelled, filled the land with forests of trees like these, the oldest of his saved species.

Over the years, Storm had watched these redwood giants stretch their limbs until now they pushed against the top of the curved dome, reaching to soar out and upward to the sky, inching, inching, ever inching to the heavens to expand, to live. It was as though the trees pleaded with him to lift the dome and free them.

It is too soon, my friends. Too soon. Without the Caplac domes you would soon die.

His father and mother had planted most of the trees; his father had started building the plastin bubbles when the glaciers started to melt, long before most people thought protection would become necessary to maintain life. Many laughed, thought his father was insane to start such a project. They felt sure the people of earth would not let their planet die.

But they were wrong.

Like the smoke from the fire, thoughts of his father hovered around him. Even as a small boy, Storm knew there was a mystery to be uncovered, a powerful reason that his father was suddenly gone. He wanted to know more about his father, everything about him, but his mother always remained silent on the subject, would only say, "It was his time." There had to be more. Storm knew there was much more to discover, to understand.

But he would have to flow with the wind, accept that the true answers to his many questions might always remain hidden from him, like the dark side of the moon.

His mind would not settle down; uncontrolled, it jumped from one thought to another. Zoe. Again!

He imagined her and her daughter happy in the domes. Would the two of them blossom to become an important part of his life?

He should step away, let her go, let her find her own path. If she were ever to find peace or happiness, she would need more time to know herself, to heal.

She would need for him to let her go, need to become unencumbered.

His gaze shifted to the sky, following the moon as it slipped from under a thick layer of clouds. Roaming, distracting thoughts continued to interfere with what had to be done.

Release!

He must untangle, free himself from all of these earthbound tentacles if he was to enter the astral plane, a place where everything and nothing were only words to be left behind. He hummed his centering note, a musical tone that signaled total focus.

The harmonic should have emptied him, allowed him to fall away and flow deeper into the great void with each releasing breath.

But his concentration still was not complete.

He had not shed his earthly skin; he still reveled in the night air that danced across his naked body, enjoyed the stretch and pull of tendons and muscles folding him into a cross-legged crouch. He felt the sudden hardness of the loamy-rich earth as he settled down.

Earth! Our Earth! Mother Earth!

His body tingled with his human senses. He tried to float away, float freely into the intense, mind-shifting meditation. His hands traced a circular pathway over the small fire.

Round and round. Again and again.

The golden light hovered, returned, allowed him to fold into something that eluded definition or borders, something that brought with it a feeling of wholeness, of oneness, an alignment with a universe both vast and unknowable.

As always, he sensed others were there; many spirits, not visible while he was still in his earthbound shell. But he knew they were there, as much a part of the golden light as he was. His soul swelled, yearned to see the others. Those who were, and those who were to be.

The fire waned; he stared into the fading embers. He scattered handfuls of fresh cedar chips, and the dying coals flashed for an instant and released a heavy, woody fragrance.

His breath took him deeper. Deeper, deeper.

Deeper into the oneness. Deeper into the all-seeing. Deeper into the everything.

Now, the light burned bright within him. The rich golden essence penetrated him through and through, leaving his head light, his eyes unfocused and filled with an inner expanding vision. The moon's silvery glow illuminated the valley stretching between him and San Francorp.

Its barrenness saddened him, as always. His mother said this stretch of land once held an abundance of trees, shrubs, and other vegetation that gave texture and life to the land. He sensed the life *still* there.

Waiting.

Earth still remained. Scarred, but fighting to live.

A rush of hope soared in his heart, reaffirming his sworn oath.

The Revivers would bring back what had been so carelessly thrown away.

He filled his lungs deeply, catching and holding onto the pleasant scent of cedar. He closed his eyes again and sifted out all thoughts and sensations that had distracted his total concentration.

Before he could release, he would have to connect with Zoe Hidalga's essence. He must know the answers. Will she live…or will she die?

The golden light filled him and swelled.

Yes! She was there. Still alive. And her child was with her. Happiness grew. Hope grew.

He reached for his panpipe and sent a haunting melody across the valley. The notes rose, lifted toward the heavens, carried his voice to the stars.

His spirit flowed with the music. It floated—rising, rising, rising, melding with the past, present, and future pathways of the woman and child.

Storm sensed their danger; saw the duality of their fate. Knew he must step away.

Her universe, as his, was filled with choices. They were hers to make. She must shape her own destiny.

She would have to accept, believe, endure. Only then would he be free to go to her.

Chapter 43

Corporit Safe House

Zoe stood over her sleeping daughter, whose presence filled her with love. She studied everything about Laya. She wanted to wake her, hug her, kiss her, breathe in her essence, tell her how much she loved her. Instead, she looked down at her long curling lashes, her dark, shining hair, and in that moment, Zoe became whole again. For the first time in two years, she could do something as fulfilling and important as simply watching her beautiful daughter breathe, watch her sleep.

Laya was finally back at her side where she belonged. Zoe vowed that she and her daughter would never separate again.

"We have to get out of here now," Zoe mumbled as she forced herself to turn away from the sleeping child.

The stabilizing patch had brought her back from the brink of death, but she still needed the chemical stimulants that were beginning to kick in. If they didn't leave, get away soon, they would be trapped and caught, torn from each other forever.

She walked to the living room. Seka and Nathan were so wrapped up in each other, they never saw her standing at the doorway.

Seated on the sofa, they held each other so tightly that they almost morphed into one human being. They were in their own separate world, lost in each other, Maybe it was the light, a contrasting eerie, soft-gray shadow, but the couple emanated a warm glowing radiance that seemed to come from nowhere and everywhere. Zoe watched Nathan pull Seka even closer, she whispered something in his ear. He gently set her at arm's length and spoke quietly in a singsong soothing voice that was seductive, and reassuring at the same time.

"The chemical enhancers have nothing to do with my love for you," he said. "You must know that by now. Know it in here." He pressed his hand over her heart. "Know it, really know it deep inside. I promise, I'll never leave you…today or tomorrow. I swear I'll be here. No one will ever keep us apart again."

"I believe you, Nathan, I really do," Seka said and exhaled a deep sigh. "But, please, can't we go now?"

"I promised Andrew I would help Zoe. She's my friend and I can't let her down." Seka hung on his every word; her eyes never left his.

Zoe was impressed by their devotion to each other.

Who can blame her for her concern? She's as frightened of losing Nathan as I am of losing Laya.

Zoe wished the two of them weren't part of this, wished she could just leave without them. Ignore them. They only complicated the situation. But Zoe was alive because of them. And it was her fault they were in this dangerous mess, and couldn't get on with their own lives.

They had to act now if they were going to survive, but at the same time, she was filled with near overwhelming indecision. Fear began to eat away at her resolve.

Doomed if she left. Doomed if she stayed.

She had only minutes to think it through, and there was no room for error. *She* would have to figure this out. The lives of Nathan, Seka, and Laya were in her hands.

Zoe stole another glance at the couple. They were still clutching each other, staring into each other's eyes.

Zoe turned away. There had to be some way, some plan that would give all of them a chance to survive. A chance to get to the Noncorp sector and Asher Wind Storm.

Zoe knew practically nothing about the various routes in and out of San Francorp. Her visit to the CARE units was the first time she had ever entered the Noncorp zone. But she did know they couldn't dare cross at any of the guarded gates. CAPOs, security forces would all be on the lookout for the four of them. And with Laya, they would stand out even more. They would need to find a way out that an eight-year-old could manage and survive.

And then it came to her. “Nathan! Seka!”

The two of them turned, startled. They moved apart like teenagers caught in some forbidden act.

“Organ Harvesting! That’s our exit to the other side. I know that building like the back of my hand,” Zoe said. “It’s not only at the far end of the city, it’s smack on the border.”

She snatched up a pencil and pad from the coffee table, then drew a diagram of the facility in bold strokes.

“I think we can get out this way,” she said, pointing at the drawing. Seka pulled away from Nathan, leaned forward to listen. Nathan eased off the sofa, went to the window, and cracked the blinds.

“The Organ Harvesting structure sits right at the edge of the Noncorp zone. It hangs over a canyon of waste. In all the years I’ve worked there, I’ve never seen any guards around it.”

“That’s right!” Seka said. “That might work.”

“You’re familiar with Organ Harvesting?” Zoe asked Nathan.

“Not particularly, but Seka worked there, too,” he said. “You’re both alumnae.” He continued to keep watch on the streets the apartment house.

The two women looked at each other and Zoe knew it was true from the grim set of Seka’s jaw.

“Dammit!” Nathan shouted.

“What’s wrong?” Zoe hurried to the window.

“Turn off the night light, Seka!” Nathan said. “Now!” The room plunged into total darkness.

“Uniformed CAPOs! Two of them. There! In the doorway on the other side of the street.”

“I knew this would happen,” Seka said.

The three of them stood side-by-side and looked down into the street.

“The last time I saw those two, they were scratching their thick heads in the Corpmall wondering where the hell I’d disappeared to,” Nathan said.

“It’s probably my fault,” Seka said. “I’m not very good at

playing cat and mouse."

"Don't blame yourself. The important thing is that we have to divert them, draw them away."

"They can't know you're here, Zoe," Nathan said. "Dutton's only suspicious of us, but there's a kill-on-sight order out on you."

"I won't let you become decoys for Laya and me."

"We have a secure telelink here," Nathan said. "Maybe we should try to get in touch with Andrew, see if he can set up a diversion."

"No!" Zoe said, shaking her head. "We can't do that! It could expose Andrew's Defy network. It might even hurt Storm. I can't risk having that happen."

"Who's Storm?" Seka asked.

"Someone you'll meet very soon … if we ever get out of here."

Zoe thought for a moment. "What if we all leave the building at the same time, split up?"

"Divide and conquer!" Seka said.

"I don't like it," Nathan said. "They'll go for Zoe and Laya and not worry about us. Too risky!"

"Okay, what if we gamble that they think only Seka is in here?" Zoe said.

"So, if I leave first," Seka said, "they'll probably follow me."

"No! I'm not letting you out of my sight," Nathan said, clutching her hand. "If you're leaving, I'm going with you."

"Okay, we'll go together," Seka said, smiling at him. She turned to Zoe. "Once you see them take off to follow us, you and Laya can slip out of here."

"And we'll meet later, in the northeast plaza," Zoe said.

"Yes … at the Nicola Flower Fountain," Seka said.

Nathan looked at his watch. "Midnight?"

"Will that give the two of you enough time?"

"If we're not there by then, don't wait for us. Just take off."

Zoe wrapped her arms around them. "The two of you have

been so wonderful. I owe you my life. There's nothing I wouldn't do for you." Tears rolled down her cheek. "I wish I could think of something else, think of a better way out of this…but I can't."

* * *

Zoe held Laya's hand in a tight grip. They stood in the darkened room, looking out the window. The CAPOs were still in a doorway across the street, talking to one another.

"Did you have a good sleep?" Zoe asked.

"Yes, but it's still night time."

"I know; I didn't want to wake you, but we have to leave soon."

"Where're we going, Mommy?"

"To the bubbles, that beautiful place I told you about."

"Is it far?"

"Very far. It may take us the rest of the night to get there." She pulled Laya close. "It's going to be a…a scary adventure. You'll have to be very brave."

Zoe saw the CAPOs stop talking and look across the street. She assumed Seka and Nathan must have left the building.

"Like when you took me away from the school?"

"Yes, sweetheart." She swallowed hard. "But we both have to be brave if we're always going to be together."

"I can do it." Laya snuggled in closer to her mother. "I won't let myself be scared."

They watched Seka and Nathan step into the street and turn, taking the opposite direction Zoe and Laya would take. The two agents looked away, pretended they weren't interested.

"Where're they going, Mommy?"

"Across town. We'll see them later." But the CAPOs still weren't taking the bait. They weren't following Nathan and Seka.

"Do you like Nathan, Mommy?"

"He's a good friend. So is Seka."

"But I mean, could he be your boyfriend?"

Despite everything going on around them, Zoe laughed.

"No, he's just a friend and he's Seka's boyfriend. Okay?"

Laya nodded and pointed toward the street. "Look, Mommy! Those men are leaving. Can go now, too?"

"Yes, but we have to be very, very careful. Zoe buttoned Laya's jacket and pulled on her own coat. At the doorway, she hesitated, knelt down, and kissed her daughter's cheek. "I'm going to need your help, Laya. Promise you'll do everything I tell you. No holding back. No questions."

Laya nodded and opened the door for them.

* * *

Mother and daughter checked to make sure the CAPOs had followed Nathan and Seka, then hurried out of the safe house and headed toward the electro-magno station. Zoe's legs were unsteady, and she fought exhaustion with every step. Laya walked by her side, clutched her hand, and seemed to be in a dream state.

Even though Zoe tried not to look back, her heart started pounding in her ears and fear forced her to turn and check to see if anyone was tailing them. For now, it looked like their plan was working. Everything seemed quiet and very normal—if anything could ever be normal again. It didn't look like they were being tracked. But when they left the safe house, Zoe knew they would become even more vulnerable to everything and anything. Walking targets! They could be shot in the back at any moment by a sharp-eyed CAPO.

She had no illusions about her worth to Corporit. She was listed for termination and they would kill her on sight. But even the vicious CAPOs wouldn't kill a child, would they?

Her stomach churned.

Yes, they would. They would kill Laya, too.

The two of them had to keep going. They had to make it for Laya's sake.

As they drew nearer to the station, there was a scattering of paid demonstrators wandering around in groups. It was common knowledge that as elections grew closer, more and more of these shills were hired to work around the clock. The voices grew even louder, more strident as they entered the electro-magno station.

Zoe and Laya eased their way through one group after another, blending and moving ahead. The closer they got to their destination, the more banners were held high in the air. And the shouting became deafening.

"Kill the Aughts! Kill the terrorists at our borders! Corporits are our friends, our protectors!"

More propaganda. More lies.

When a pod arrived, Zoe searched the faces of all the people who boarded at the same time. Everyone looked grim and tired; none of them looked suspicious. These were the people who worked the off-hour shifts for departments that needed twenty-four hour coverage. None of them seemed to have any interest in her and Laya. By the time they arrived at their destination, the pod had very few passengers.

Chapter 44

Organ Harvesting Plaza
Nicola Flower Fountain

The Nicola Flower Fountain and the surrounding plaza were dead ahead. Zoe and Laya sat on the ground, alert and watchful. They had just finished another perimeter search of the area, but everything seemed to be deserted. No movement, no sign of life.

The silence was nerve-wracking.

Zoe eyed the Organ Harvest building next to the plaza. It was like an evil apparition against the moonlit skyline, a monstrous predator ready to strike.

She planned to hide them inside the fountain to avoid being spotted by any stray patrolling units. But to get to the fountain, they would have to dodge the knee-high stone benches where Zoe had spent many lunchtimes. It was one of very few fountains still allowed to operate—this one a sop for the organ harvesters—but at this hour, the fountain's water was turned off to help preserve the precious resource.

Laya whispered in Zoe's ear, "Where are Seka and Nathan?"

"They'll be here soon."

"Mommy, do you like Seka?"

"I like her a lot," Zoe said. "And I'm very grateful to her. She saved my life."

"Will she be my aunt when we get to the other place?"

"You know, Laya. I think she'd be honored to have you as a niece. Anyone would."

Zoe was only half-listening to Laya, distracted by their circumstances. It was dangerous for them to be out in the open like this, but it would be even worse when they had to travel across the open park to the fountain. And they had to do it soon—a patrol could spot them at any time, suddenly and without warning.

Just do it!

She grabbed Laya's hand and they ran to the fountain, climbed up and squeezed between the iridescent metallic petals that rose ten feet in the air. They dropped down into the center where it was still damp from having gushed water most of the day.

It was the perfect place to hide. And it was the only place.

Earlier, the sky had been thick with haze. Now, strangely, the sky was crystal clear.

Nights like this were rare; a heavy atmosphere was more what Zoe had expected. She watched the moon float freely, casting a silvery light. It made the Nicola sculpture glow with an effervescent sparkle; stars dotted the sky, and everything seemed peaceful. Beautiful.

Beautiful...and dangerous!

She peeked at the clock on the fifth floor façade of the Organ Harvesting building. Time passed and she grew edgier. Seka and Nathan were twenty minutes late for the midnight meet.

They should have left already. Can't wait much longer.

Zoe had vowed to get her daughter to a safe place and she intended to do exactly that. But Nathan and Seka had saved her life. How could she just leave them?

We're all helpless, destined to be caught in a CAPO trap at any moment.

No! She could not leave just yet. She had to wait for them a little longer.

Zoe needed to do something to distract the both of them. She nudged Laya and pointed to different constellations. "See the three stars in a row? Do you know what they're called?"

Laya pointed at the sky along with her mother and shook her head. "No, Mommy."

"That's Orion's belt. He's a giant that lives in the sky."

"I see it."

"And all those tiny little stars bunched together? That's the

Seven Sisters."

"It's like a big story book hanging right above us."

Zoe, laughed. "You're right…I never thought of it like that. But all the constellations tell a story."

The diversion kept the two of them occupied, and calmed them. Zoe's breath caught. Storm was there, among the stars.

"What's wrong, Mommy?"

A shiver of pleasure tickled her spine. "It's nothing. I thought I heard something."

She stared at the wispy image of Storm, waited for Laya to see him, too. But the vision was only there for Zoe.

She remembered the first time his face had appeared to her at the safe house, and now, he was here again, so clear, so real. How much her life had changed since that first brief encounter.

"What do you see, Mommy?"

"There!" she said, pointing to a bright star that glittered in Storm's right eye. "That's the North Star. We'll use it to guide us."

"Will it take us long to get to the bubbles, the place with the beautiful trees?" Laya asked, snuggling closer.

Zoe squeezed her daughter, then fingered the stabilizer patch that clung to her shoulder.

"Let's hope not." She glanced up at the clock again.

Where are they? They should have been here long ago.

"It feels creepy in here," Laya whispered. "I wish Seka and Nathan would hurry."

"Me, too, sweetheart." Zoe ran her fingers through her daughter's curly hair and caressed her soft cheeks. "But it won't be long now." She gave Laya a tight hug and surrendered to the moment, the joy of just holding her child.

An inner glow of happiness gave way to an overwhelming sense of peace.

* * *

A distant scream of sirens shattered the silence, brought Zoe back to the moment. Nathan and Seka were now more than thirty minutes late.

She could visualize the drawing she'd made at the safe house; she mentally reviewed the plan. Could she carry it off alone? The VMAS cloud had lifted, replaced by her strength and resolve.

The wailing sirens grew closer.

"We have to leave, now!" she whispered to Laya.

A hand clamped down on Zoe's shoulder. She jumped up, spun around, fists ready to fight.

"It's us," Seka said quietly.

Zoe's breathing was loud, ragged. "I almost left without you. The sirens? Are they for you?"

"They're right behind us," Nathan screamed above the noise. "We couldn't get away from them. We tried, but we must have brought them here. Dammit, I knew we shouldn't have come. I didn't know what else to do, where to go."

"Let's just get out of here!" Zoe shouted.

Nathan scooped up Laya and they ran toward the Organ Harvesting building. Zoe led them around the side to an auxiliary entrance; she pressed two fingers against the DNA sensor.

Nothing.

"Shit! I'm locked out of the system. I should have thought of that."

"Let me try!" Seka said. "I may still have access."

The door swished open just as the first CAPO hovervan turned into the Organ Harvesting compound. But they were in.

The air lock whooshed closed behind the four of them; instantly cutting off the blare of the CAPO sirens.

Nathan flinched like he'd hit a wall. "My God! What's that stench?" He covered his mouth and nose, coughed harshly.

"Human rot." Zoe said in a flat voice.

She led them down through a blue-lit corridor, between a maze of cables and clear tubing carrying cloudy, amorphous fluids. Their shadows fused into a single blob on the metallic walls.

As they walked, the stench grew even stronger; Zoe's nostrils felt like they were on fire, she assumed the others were having the same problem.

"I can't breathe, Mommy," Laya said, gagging.

Nathan took Seka's scarf and wrapped it around Laya's face. "How could the two of you stand to work here day after day?" His voice had a tinny sound; he clutched at his chest, turned, and vomited.

* * *

A rush of voices echoed through the corridor ahead of them. "Dammit!" Seka said. "They're in the building already."

"This way!" Zoe turned into an offshoot from the main corridor that led them down a small passageway. They stooped until they were almost bent in half, but they still kept banging their heads against the overhead.

"Where we going?" Nathan whispered. "This is suffocating. I can't stand this much longer."

"Up ahead!"

A miniature doorway led them into a massive, ten-story rotunda, so brightly lit it blinded them. The odor was so vile in the huge enclosure it became a malignant presence that crawled down the throat, strangled.

When their eyes adjusted to the lights, Nathan was stunned, frozen in place.

All around them were huge glass tanks filled with a bubbling, translucent fluid. In the center of each container, the solution washed over the skinless body of a man, or woman, or child. All were spiked with multiple tubes that bit into their flesh like clinging vipers.

"Oh, my God!" Nathan choked out. He pressed Laya's face into his shoulder.

Zoe and Seka were silent.

Nathan's eyes remained wide open, unblinking, as though he couldn't stop himself from taking in the surreal horrors around him. Before Zoe could stop him, he dipped a hand into the nearest tank and touched a floating arm. Eyelids snapped open; empty sockets gaped back.

Nathan stumbled backwards, crashing hard into another

tank; fluid splashed out on and around him.

"My God, they're alive!"

"This," Seka said, "is what I couldn't tell you."

"Why would they do this? Keep people alive, stored in tanks?"

"The tanks preserve the organs until the dissection process is almost completed," Zoe said. "They've developed a near-perfect way to keep living tissue nourished and viable."

Nathan's mouth opened, he tried to speak, but the words refused to come.

"It's cost-effective," Seka said and pointed upward. "The seventh level looks exactly like this one. I worked in a laboratory close by until—"

"Stop it! Don't torture yourself!" Zoe said, squeezing her arm.

But Seka couldn't stop. "Preserving arteries was my specialty. Other specialists stripped the non-vitals; first eyes, then ears, digits, limbs, skin. All the time keeping them alive until there was nothing of value except the internal organs and vessels."

"After they were taken off viability support and euthanized, I got them," Zoe said. "I cut away, dissected, and preserved the organs…and whatever else was useable … before electronic cremation of the remains."

"Is this what the Corporit culture is really about?" Nathan asked. "Putting living beings into tanks? Why would any civilized society do this to human beings?"

"Our numbers have kept growing smaller while our needs grew greater," Zoe said. "Simple as that."

"At first, it was larger and more ambitious research projects that demanded more and more bodies," Seka said, her voice clipped and tight. "But as they refined advanced biogenetic techniques, keeping, and then using these people, became a permanent way of storing organs and body parts for implantation for the privileged. It was also the prize of immortality for the obedient or for those who chose the right political direction."

"The final step was to further tailor their corruption," Zoe said, "so DPs, Defys, and political enemies of the system would undergo a final, torturous punishment. This is what awaited those who defied the Corporit system."

"There's so many of them," Nathan said, looking up at the circular scaffold-like structure. Layer upon layer of preservation tanks filled every available inch of the vast arena, from the base level where they stood, to the top of the ten-story building.

Suspended in the center was a huge mother unit from which nutrient-filled tubes snaked out, piercing and surrounding each tank-housed body.

"Corporit science at work," Zoe said.

"Murderous bastards! This is what was my job was really about. What Dutton never told explained to me." Nathan was obviously stunned; his face turned a ghastly white. "Not just population control or salvageable body parts, but a form of immortality as a corporate prize for the privileged and the compliant. And *I* was the one in charge of perpetuating these horrors."

"Some of these poor people have been attached to this support system for years, waiting until their particular cells are needed," Zoe said.

"And you have no idea," Seka said, "what hell it is when the computers or the machinery fouls up and all these sedated zombies start flopping around, trying to yank out their tubes and free themselves." She covered her face.

"I'm so sorry," Nathan whispered.

* * *

"Doctor Quinn!" boomed a deep voice boomed over the in-house telespeaker. "This is Emory Dutton. This nonsense has gone far enough. Do not attempt to run! We know where you are."

Zoe, Laya, Nathan, and Seka huddled tightly together. The only sound was the hypnotic on-again, off-again thump of the life-support machinery echoing through the vast facility. Nathan untangled Laya's arms from around his neck and stood her next to Zoe. "I'll turn myself in. It's me he's after. He might not even know you and Seka are here."

"Forget whatever it is you're thinking," Zoe said. "He knows who's here. Security identified us the moment we entered the building. He may have called out your name, but don't think for a moment he's going to allow *any* of us to go. He probably doesn't know exactly where we are right now, but that will change fast. We've got to keep moving if we're going to have any chance of getting away."

They remained together, but no one moved. "There's no way out," Dutton announced.

Zoe's mind started to wander, then she realized what was happening: Paralyzing sonic waves had started pulsating through their brains, scrambling their neural receptors. They stood stiff-legged with unfocused eyes, caught in the rhythm of the soundless pulsations.

Fading in and out of a timeless euphoria, Zoe's mind was slowing down. She looked at Laya. The scarf was still wrapped around her head.

Focus! Got to focus!

She was at the domes. They were all at the domes. She could visualize them there. Safe.

Happy. Zoe held onto the vision.

"Seka! Nathan!" she said, tugging at their arms.

* * *

A loud voice boomed throughout the building. "There's an energy drain in one of the probes, Mr. Dutton. It's not holding the sonic wave; it's dissipating."

"Potek!" Dutton yelled. "Get that probe online again. Now!"

"I'm trying, sir. It's not responding."

The two voices continued to broadcast over the telespeaker. "Get the hell down there," Dutton screamed. "Find them. Secure them! Now! We can't let them get away, damn it!"

* * *

Zoe's breath caught. She clutched Laya's hand and stared

at her friends. Their arms were outstretched, still trapped by the synaptic freeze.

She got behind Seka and pushed her until she began to walk on her own, slowly and in the right direction. Grabbing Nathan's wrist and clutching Laya, she caught up with Seka and guided the three of them to an emergency exit. Ready to push though, she stopped and looked back.

She would have to disable the emergency door alarm system or the CAPOs would locate them right away.

"Next level!" came a voice from above. Zoe realized they were systematically checking each level.

Frantic, she searched wildly, trying to find something that would kill the alarms. A switch, a valve.

"I don't see them, Commander!"

"I'm on my way. Try the other side."

Zoe backed away, bumped into a tank as she looked around. She stared at the bobbing body; its empty sockets looked back at her. It was as if it could see her, know who she was, follow her movements. Wincing, she sank her arm into the tank and yanked the tubes out.

A klaxon immediately broadcast the disconnect.

Zoe dashed from tank to tank, pulling out every tube she could get her hands on, then made her way back to where she'd left Laya, Nathan, and Seka. Each disconnect had tripped an additional alarm. The nerve-shattering cacophony drowned out the sound of the emergency door alarm when she opened the portal and pushed the three of them through.

She bolted the door behind them.

Chapter 45

Dutton and Potek stood on the tenth-floor observation deck of the Organ Harvest rotunda, overlooking the sea of tanks filled with future body parts. That's how Dutton thought of them.

Body parts. Sort of like when mechanics had a stash of cannibalized pieces from broken vehicles that were otherwise of no value to anyone. Spare parts.

He studied a nearby tank. Whatever was in there bore no resemblance to any real person.

Armless, legless, even its nipples had been lopped off. Dutton turned away in disgust when its mouth started sucking on the walls of the container.

Many of his "friends" were still alive only because they were in his sphere of influence.

Otherwise, they would have been dissected and vaporized long ago. Standing there, looking down at floor after floor of these body parts, a flash of a few of his mistresses' and ex-friends' faces popped into his head. They were probably floating below somewhere with empty eye sockets, also sucking on the plastin tanks.

A chuckle of satisfaction gurgled deep in his throat.

No wonder I'm a favored dinner guest.

And he was vain enough to enjoy the lavish amounts of attention, the fawning, the brown-nosing, the ass-kissing everyone gave him.

Nothing could describe the extreme satisfaction he got from looking at those individuals who were still walking around because of his interventions. The beauty of it: after saving their necks, he had them under his thumb forever. He could ask for anything and they would do it…without hesitation. He owned them. And sooner or later, every last one of them would be asked to honor that lifesaving debt; they did not have to be reminded of those floating in the organ preservation tanks.

Oh, yes! The mere act of canceling someone's pending

execution, giving them back their tomorrows, that's the ultimate power trip.

He stared at the mother teat hanging in the center of the rotunda. Mother teat! He relished that designation.

After all, it was a massive nutrient provider, doling out life-sustaining fluids to every single tank, every single body in the place. No teat-sucking, death. Not instantly, of course.

Actually, he was told it was pretty horrible to watch. He'd elected not to do that. But they still died whether he watched or not.

The flopping tubes from the bag looked like spaghetti gone wild. The image tickled his fancy: A huge sac with hanging, fluid-filled noodles slipping and sliding over and under each other like a full-blown pasta frenzy. And who did this spaghetti dinner go to? Some asshole who had given Corporit some kind of trouble. Real or imagined.

Well, fuck them. At least these losers are good for something.

And down there somewhere were those traitors; Nathan Quinn and his slut Seka Joraine, along with the pain-in-the-ass Hidalga woman.

They'll be good for something, too.

None of these thoughts settled him the way they usually did. Disturbing questions kept buzzing in his head.

Why is this Zoe Hidalga with Quinn and Joraine? Potek told me VMAS should have finished her off, just as it did that miserable husband of hers. And the child, Laya Hidalga, was kidnapped from her school in broad daylight by her mother. Her mother! Preposterous! What's the world coming? People don't seem to know their place anymore.

"Has the neural probe been fixed yet, Potek?"

"The bodies in the tanks must have interfered with the neural penetration."

"Always some excuse! Always some lame excuse." Dutton looked over the protective railing, tried to spot one of the four fugitives that were somewhere below.

Potek remained silent.

"We both know Hidalga should have been disposed of by now. Isn't it your fault she wasn't taken into custody at her apartment?"

Potek did not respond.

"Isn't it your fault your surveillance team didn't catch up to those other two—Quinn and Joraine?"

Silence.

"Where's the 'no sir', the 'yes sir' now?" Dutton waited a beat. "And how idiotically simple is it to figure out a mother would try anything to regain her child?" Dutton bent closer to the CAPO commander, looked directly into his eyes. "You really are stupid, aren't you?"

"Yes sir."

Dutton turned his back on Potek, reached for the facility communicator. "Dr. Quinn, Dr. Joraine. Give yourselves up now and I promise we will reduce the charges against you. And Dr. Hidalga, you will get the best medical treatment available. I promise."

"Sir, I don't think they believe you."

"Of course they don't, but do you have a better idea?"

"I do, sir."

A blasting klaxon vibrated throughout the rotunda. Emory Dutton covered his ears.

Potek stood at attention, waiting to speak.

"And your plan, Commander?"

Potek screamed over the deafening sound. "Hunt them down and kill them!"

Chapter 46

Almost from the moment the metal security exit door closed behind them, Laya, Seka, and Nathan started to awaken from their stupor. The sonic waves that had scrambled their thoughts were now blocked, left behind in the main rotunda.

The four of them stood on a small landing at the bottom step of a steep spiral staircase.

Each of the risers was illuminated by dim, red emergency lights that blinked on and off. With no railing, it looked surreal, like an architectural sculpture suspended in space—a foundationless free form that climbed up and out of sight.

"I can't believe they would do this to us," Nathan said, pointing to the exit door they'd just come through. "Sonic detention is only supposed to be used on dangerous felons."

"Isn't that what we are?" Zoe said. She looked up at the floating staircase, wondered how they could get to the top without falling off. "Isn't that how the Corporits see us? Think about what we've learned, how we could expose their plot to manipulate VMAS to downsize the population…how everyone has been lied to."

"Who would believe us?" Seka said, taking Nathan's hand.

Laya stood tall next to Zoe, trying to be grown up and brave. But she looked up at Zoe with large frightened eyes.

"Face it!" Zoe said. "Our only hope is to climb up and out of here. Do it before the CAPOs pinpoint our exact location and surround us."

She moved toward the base of the staircase. "There's nothing we can do to stop them. They're untouchable! Even to think we might be able to bring them down is pure fantasy." Zoe shifted from one foot to another, trying not to scream at them. "Don't you get it? They have the upper hand. Our only chance is to escape into the Noncorp area. And if we don't get moving, get out of here right now, it'll be *us* floating, rotting in those tanks."

"You're right, Zoe," Seka said. "It shouldn't take them

long to realize that we've left the first floor tank area. And the only place we could possibly be is in one of the emergency exits."

"Well, let's get the hell out of here before they pinpoint us!" Nathan said.

They started up the spiral stairway, single file, each foot carefully placed in the center of each metal step. Just as they adjusted to the awkward climb, the emergency lights flickered out.

Their breaths merged into one loud gasp.

"Damn them!" Nathan said. "They know we're in one of the escape shafts."

Laya began to cry, tugged at Zoe's leg. "I'm scared, Mommy … there's nothing to hold onto. I'm going to fall."

"No you won't fall; I won't let you." She put a hand on the next step ahead of her, steadied herself, and reached back. "Here, take my hand."

Zoe squeezed Laya's hand; it seemed to quiet her for a moment. "Let's hope it'll take them some time discover which shaft we're in," she said to the others.

"I don't like this," Seka said, her voice shaky and small. "It's so dark. I can't see a thing."

"I'm here with you," Nathan said. "I'll hold onto you."

"But it's so black. How long do you think we'll be in here?"

"Just keep moving!" Zoe yelled.

They started climbing again, slowly. "We'll be trapped," Seka said. "That, or we'll all go flying off this thing."

"No! There's a way out…if we can get to it." Zoe was breathless. A sudden dizziness caused her foot to slip off the edge of the next step. The lurch threw her off balance. She wobbled on one foot. Laya hung onto her, tried to pull her back.

"Help me!" Laya screamed. "Mommy's going to fall!"

Seka moved up next to Laya, caught Zoe's waistband, and steadied her until both of Zoe's feet were back on the same step.

"Are you all okay?" Nathan shouted. He climbed a couple

of steps until he had a hand on Seka again.

"Yes," Zoe called back. She refused to think about anything except getting out. "But we need to keep moving. They'll be here soon."

As they started up again, Seka whispered, "I'm not going to make it!"

"Yes, you can," Laya said. "You saved my mommy…you can do anything. I'll help you. Hold onto me."

Zoe was still shaken, but she had to keep urging them on. It took all of her focus not to think about their predicament: trapped in an Organ Harvesting stairway virtually suspended in air. She couldn't afford another slip; it might tumble them all into nothingness.

"Are you counting the levels?" Zoe called out to Nathan.

"We just passed Level Six."

"Good! My count also."

Zoe tried to listen for the CAPOs, but all she heard was everyone's gasping breath—the grunts and groans became louder and louder. Laya's hand was now wet and slippery. Zoe winced every time she heard the sound of a foot slipping off a step, or the pained cry when someone skinned a shin against the unforgiving metal. She knew their muscles were weakening, starting to cramp, begging to stop.

"Only one more flight," Nathan called out.

"Hold it!" Zoe shouted.

"What is it?"

"Look down! Do you see it?"

A thin, powerful beam of yellow light was working its way up the shaft, crisscrossing, searching the open space.

"What the hell is that?" Nathan said.

"Search laser," Seka said. "If that beam touches any one of us, they'll immediately know our exact location."

"Hurry!" Zoe shouted. "Let's get to the tenth-floor exit panel!"

She could see the beam shooting higher and higher. She desperately wanted to move faster, even run, but it was too dangerous.

"Do you see the exit door, yet?" Nathan shouted.

"Yes, I'm there now, at the top."

"Remember, you have to push both release buttons at the same time," Seka said. "They're flush with the door panel."

"I know, but I can only find one of them."

"Seka!" Nathan shouted "Help her! You're the closest."

"No! I can't! I'll fall."

The beam now shone less than two floors beneath them. Zoe could hear the pleading in Nathan's voice.

"It's all right," he said. "Let me climb past you."

"No! You'll knock us off the steps. We'll fall. Die!"

"Seka, it's all right. Let go of my arm. It'll be okay."

"I'm sorry," Seka said, sobbing. "Go."

Nathan reached Zoe's side on the platform. "I've done this once before," she said, "but I can't remember where the second release button is." She tried to visualize the escape training procedures manual. "I think it's going to take the two of us to make it work."

She took his hand and guided it to the button she'd found. "You hold this one, I'll look for the other one."

His breath was hot and moist on her cheek as she started her search for the other button. A quick glance below and she could see the search laser exploring at the ninth level. Her sweaty fingers slid along the seamless metal wall, up and down, then sideways. Then she found it, the barely perceptible indentation for the second release button.

The beam was now within a few steps of Seka.

"On my count, push!" she said, taking a deep breath. "One, two, three!" They pushed, but the door didn't budge.

"Let's do it again. Only this time, I'll hold the buttons and you put everything behind your shoulder."

The beam was a foot away from Seka.

"Move up the steps," Zoe shouted. "Laya, make room for Seka! Move up onto the platform!"

"Okay, Nathan. Now! Push! Hard!"

The escape hatch popped open, tumbling the two of them into a passageway.

Zoe and Nathan reached back to pull Laya and Seka inside. Just when they thought they were in the clear, the laser beam hit Seka's foot as she was pulling it through the hatch.

An alarm shrieked. “Move!” Zoe screamed.

They raced away from the escape hatch and down a corridor; security doors clanked closed behind them.

“This way!” Zoe screamed, turning into a small laboratory. The air-lock entry mechanism clamped shut behind them.

They were now trapped inside.

Chapter 47

"Got you, you miserable traitors!" Emory Dutton rubbed his hands together and turned to Potek. "So, a successful hunt after all."

"As expected, sir."

"Maybe so," the CEO said. "I was beginning to think you didn't have the spine to get this kind of job done." He turned and gave Potek an almost-smile. "Still, you did come through, Commander." Dutton gave Potek a rare pat on the shoulder. "I'll make sure this goes on your Corporit Personnel record. Undoubtedly, this could mean more money for you. Maybe even an apartment upgrade."

Potek smiled back at him, then grinned like some old lap dog who'd just been given a treat.

"Now we have the four of them exactly where we want them." He barked out a laugh. "Like rats in a trap; they're not going anywhere locked-down in *that* laboratory. It's the end of the line for them. They're finished."

They started walking casually down corridor after corridor, edging their way to the north end of the tenth floor. Dutton wasn't in any hurry now. No, he was savoring the moment, trying to make it last as long as possible.

A winner again.

He saw that the whole escapade could work to his advantage, perhaps in ways he'd only dreamed about. Not for one moment had he actually believed he would ever be the one to bring down Rebecca and Tris Quinn...until Nathan Quinn fell into his lap.

Nothing like a good plan.

Others had tried and failed to discredit the Quinn husband-and-wife team that had influenced almost every level of medical Corporit philosophy for the past three decades. They'd stood in the way of far too many projects Dutton had tried to ramrod past the Medicorp ethics committee. With them out of the picture, there weren't too many who would stand up for the Quinns' philosophy on healthcare.

And a weak philosophy at that. Why better healthcare for the poorer individuals in our Corporit society? What have the masses ever done for society? All they do is take, take, take. Just a lot of borderline, soon to be homeless nothings dumped into the Noncorp areas. A big waste of time and money.

That he, Emory Dutton, could permanently blacken that stellar Quinn reputation and maybe even pluck and dispose of the whole lot of them, would be an incredible personal victory.

And that pissant Nathan Quinn?

He had given Dutton nothing but trouble from the first moment he stepped into the role of Desisto Chief.

But after all, he is a Quinn. A man who's never had the stones or the vision to do what needs to be done. Too much like his parents...healers instead of Corporit leaders.

Those days were over.

The CEO stopped, reached into his pocket, and pulled out his personal recorder. He brought the miniaturized speaker to his lips and dictated the future arrest orders for the Quinns.

Let's see how they hold up to interrogation when I finally bring them in.

The sudden halt surprised Potek and his team of ten. They bumped into each other to keep from knocking down the Medicorp CEO.

Dutton spoke into the tiny speaker of the recorder for a moment, then put it back into his pocket.

The actual arrest of the Quinns would have to wait, at least until he had Nathan Quinn put through interrogation. By the time Dutton got through with him, he'd confess to anything Dutton wanted. And wait until he got his hands on that traitor Seka Joraine.

That bitch will pay. She thought Organ Harvesting was a nightmare. Wait until she sees what it's like to crawl into one of the specimen tanks. No pre-sedation for her. Let's give her some time to think about what it means to cross me.

Still, he'd take no chances. He would have to get a solid confession from Nathan Quinn or incarceration of the elder Quinns would not be guaranteed. They had enough personal wealth and influence to save their miserable necks; they could even turn things around and cause Dutton a lot of problems.

Yes, I'll definitely need that confession or it will be a stand-off.

"Take a good look at this escapade, Potek. It's a perfect example of why the Corporits run the world with such success."

"I don't understand, sir."

"Of course you don't." Dutton smiled benignly at the commander. "And that's why you'll always be in some subservient position."

Potek remained silent.

Dutton noticed the commander wasn't smiling this time. "Let me enlighten you, Potek."

Dutton treasured these moments. When you could slow down time and revel in an act of accomplishment, turn it into a large palpable feast.

"These misfits we've cornered in that stinking laboratory," Dutton said, on the move again. "Why do you think they're about to go down?"

The CEO looked at the silent commander, waited a click for a response, then said, "It's really pretty simple—they don't know how to plan. Unless you call being trapped in some dumb, organ slave pit a plan."

"Not much of a plan, sir."

"That's right, Potek. And that's the quality of thinking you get from the Noncorps and people who think life, or our existence, is an evolving utopian masterpiece."

"I'm not sure—"

Dutton stopped again, this time in front of a specimen tank. A floating female rolled, looked toward him with unseeing eyes. A momentary spike of revulsion took hold as he looked inside the tank. All the musculature of her legs had been stripped away; from the groin down, she was nothing but a skeleton.

“Political daydreamers. That’s what they are.” Dutton’s voice was rising. “That’s why when governments collapsed around the globe, Corporit was in the wings, ready and able to absorb them, or reduce those that still remained to virtual non-existence.”

“Yes sir.”

“It’s not as though everything just falls into place, Commander. Democracy is an ideal, but it doesn’t assure happiness. Do you understand that, Potek?”

“I think so, sir.”

“People want to be shown the way. The best way. They’re like children. They don’t really know what’s good for them. Tell them what to do and they feel secure and useful.

Anything else fosters confusion and dissatisfaction.”

“Yes sir.”

“The corporations were good planners. They planned every step of the takeover,” Dutton said. “Planning. That’s why we won the Corporit wars.”

“Yes sir.”

“Do Nathan Quinn, his slut Seka Joraine, and this Zoe Hidalga and her spawn, even know what they’re running to?”

“My impression is they were trying to get to the Noncorp zone.”

“And they would have fit right in.” Dutton laughed and looked at his buffed nails. “Noncorps are dreamers, Potek, just like the four people trapped inside that lab. The kind of riff- raff, the idiots who don’t have a p-l-a-n.”

“Yes sir.”

Chapter 48

Zoe knew this lab all too well. She went to a cubicle and looked at her former workspace, wondered how she'd endured being there day after day.

Nathan didn't follow her, but prowled the laboratory like a trapped animal. Agitated, restless, caged.

Zoe, Seka, and Laya watched him check the length and width of the room, slink in and out of cubicles, circle the worktables.

He stopped in front of the laboratory's massive collection of knives. The instruments were meticulously lined up according to size and function. Each of them was sharp, clean, and ready to dissect human tissue.

Nathan's face drained of color. Zoe thought he might pass out. But he jerked away from looking at the tools to study the expanse of the ceiling in the windowless enclosure. Without warning, he smashed his fist into a wall and instantly cried out, shaking his hand frantically to ease the pain.

"These are solid," he choked out. "There's no way out of here. That bastard Dutton nailed us. We're finished."

"It's not over," Zoe said. "I've worked here for the past two years; I know every inch of this lab. There's still a chance."

Nathan didn't seem to hear her; he shuffled around aimlessly, in a daze. He stopped in front of several small holding tanks. Groups of eviscerated organs were squeezed together, piled one on top of the other. Preservatives had mutated them into a ghastly bright orange, more like an extraterrestrial's viscera than anything human.

Although the entire laboratory was spotless, chemically cleaned, and sterilized, the penetrating acrid aroma of preserving solution reached out like creeping tentacles everywhere. It strangled all of them. Zoe knew every breath she took was laced with the unmistakable stench of death.

Her eyes tracked the intricate network of a stainless steel

conveyor belt that stretched out and crawled through the entire length and breadth of the room, connecting all of the dissection tables to a single central spine. It terminated at a large vacuum-locked, see-through unit. All eyes followed Zoe's.

"That's the disintegration chamber," Zoe said. They all focused on it.

"Thank you, doctors!" a voice boomed from the overhead telespeaker. The four of them froze.

"How ironic you found this particular spot. I want to thank you for making this so convenient," the voice continued, drawing out each word in a noxious tone. "You couldn't have chosen a more appropriate place to end this ridiculous rebellion. You'll either do as I say right now, or you're all dead."

"It's Dutton!" Seka said.

"What the hell's he talking about?" Nathan said.

Laya grabbed her mother's hand; her dark eyes were large and frightened. "Mommy, that man sounds mean."

"It's his warped way of reminding us that the entire lab becomes a bio-disintegration chamber if he activates the destruct sequence," Zoe said. "Any organic material in this laboratory will be reduced to ashes almost instantly."

"The bastard's right. From his prospective it is ironic," Seka said. She turned to face Nathan. "The system was designed to deal with biological accidents and contamination…or to destroy unusually large amounts of useless tissue."

Dutton's voice attacked them again. "Think about it! You have the option of walking out of there alive, or being vaporized. There is still a way to settle this without anyone dying. Just give yourselves up."

After a very brief pause, Dutton continued. "I wish I could say, we'll kiss and make up, or all is forgiven and your old jobs will be waiting for you. But we all know that would be a lie. Still, whatever you face will be a lot better than disintegrating. Don't you agree?"

Dutton's humorless chuckle filled the room. "Not much of a choice, I'll grant you. But that's it. Take it or leave it. And Dr.

Quinn, do think of your mother and father. Think of what this will mean to them to lose their only son. This whole escapade could even ruin them, destroy their futures."

Nathan looked directly into the camera. "Shut up, Dutton. You can't do anything to my parents. You'd have wiped them out a long time ago if you could have gotten away with it. It took me a long time to figure that out."

"Yes, Dr. Quinn, you've been too spoiled and coddled to understand much of anything about the *real* Corporit world." His voice was filled with venom. "But no one is untouchable, Dr. Quinn. Not even your noble family."

Nathan's face flushed in anger, but he remained silent.

"Dr. Hidalga, think this over very carefully. If you walk out now, your child will never have to contract VMAS. We now have a vaccine, and we can provide you with a VMAS stabilizer."

"Liar!" Zoe shouted. "You'll murder me along with everyone else."

"And your child?" Dutton shouted. "What about her? What about *her* future? You risked her life to take her out of the school…all because you were selfish, wanted her at your side.

Wouldn't she have been better off in the orphanage school rather than facing death? Think about it. Do you really want me to start the contamination countdown with her in there? Do you want her to die?"

"Don't listen to him, Zoe," Nathan said. "We're just *things* to him. Useless. That's the way that maniac thinks." Nathan wrapped an arm around Seka and pulled her to him. "If we walk out that door, Dutton's going to kill us. I'd rather die right here than fall into his hands. Zoe, How long do we have?"

Zoe moved quickly across the room. "There's a countdown safety procedure to allow personnel enough time to evacuate." She slammed her hand against a button-switch.

Silently, the conveyor began to move toward the closed disintegration chamber. The door's vacuum seal popped, gave way, and whooshed open.

Zoe plunged her arms into the nearest tank and started flinging out hearts, livers, lungs, kidneys, pancreas, blobs of saved connective tissue, and any other odds and ends she could grab. She threw all of it onto the stainless steel belt. The entire room became an organ-filled, canvas in splattered orange.

The belt continued its journey; it moved through the room like a lazy snake toting throwaway human tissue on its back, crawling steadily toward its destination—the disintegration chamber.

"Help me!" she shouted. "We need this stuff to get us out of here!"

Seka joined in. Nathan and Laya hesitated, then started by picking up organs, first delicately, but after a moment, more hurriedly, flinging them onto the belt.

"Clever!" Dutton said. "But it's not going to do you any good. You'll never make it. You're all going to die right where you stand! Dr. Quinn, this is your last chance. All of you walk toward the door…or it's all over."

Zoe glanced at the nearest surveillance camera and quickened her pace.

"So you want to make a race out of it?" Dutton's harsh voice, all pretense of its earlier humor gone, blasted throughout the laboratory. "Good!"

Crimson warning lights began to flash; the eerie wail of a siren echoed off the walls, surrounded them.

"How long now?" Nathan said.

"I don't know," Zoe said. "Depends on where he's set the controls. Anything from thirty seconds to two minutes."

The variety of organs and body pieces slid into the chamber, their weight registering on a digital read-out.

"We need forty-five kilograms to activate the disintegration process in the chamber," yelled Zoe. She reached for a heart and tossed it toward the chamber. Erratically, the heart bounced on the belt like a ball and finally dropped into the chamber, registering the required mass.

The conveyors stopped, a gong and a hiss announced the

closing of the vacuum-sealed unit, sealing the orange pile of human organs inside.

A rapid series of lights flashed the progress of the program. Within seconds, they watched the mass of material reduce to a small pile of ashes. When the outside doors opened, high-powered fans drove the ashes out of the disintegrator into a huge descending debris chute.

"Twenty seconds!" Zoe shouted, standing by the chamber. "That's all we've got before the chamber regenerates. After that, our weight will retrigger the ignition system. We've got to pass through the disintegrator to the other side and out to the chute before it closes again. That's our way out. Our only way out!"

The door swished open and the conveyor began to move.

"Take Laya with you!" Zoe yelled to Nathan, knocking approaching organs off the conveyor to prevent them from entering the chamber.

"No, Mommy. I won't go without you. Not without you."

"Get out of here!" both Nathan and Seka yelled at Zoe. "Now!"

Nathan screamed. "Don't argue!"

Zoe grabbed Laya and pushed her into the chamber.

"Move!" she yelled, shoving Laya's backside until there was enough room for her to crawl through also.

When they were both through the chamber and on the outside, at the edge of the vertical chute, Zoe looked back, barely caught the words of another Dutton taunt from inside the lab.

"—time's running out!"

Seka pushed Nathan inside the chamber ahead of her. "We can't both get through there at the same time."

The conveyors stopped.

"Remember?" Nathan shouted. "I said I wasn't going anywhere without you!" He jumped back into the lab and grabbed her hand.

* * *

Dutton glanced at the automatic sequence panel playing out its rapid, methodical step-by- step functions. It irked him that

Hidalga and her daughter were outside of the lab. The chance that they could get away represented failure. It would show vulnerability.

He needed to capture them, have them in hand.

But they weren't going anywhere. There was no real escape. He'd approved the original plans of the dump chute and he knew it took a sharp quarter mile dive straight down the side of a cliff. If they dropped into it, they were dead anyway.

She and that child are nothing, but they belong in custody. That's what our system requires. Control. Corporit control. Everyone has to live by the rules. My rules. But, dammit, I want Nathan Quinn. He is the real prize here.

He watched Quinn and Joraine. They wrapped their arms around each other, squeezed together, fused into one. As they kissed, the disintegration chamber's doors slammed shut and a blinding flash filled the laboratory. All living tissue was transformed into residual ashes. Dutton stared at the empty room.

That's how we deal with traitors, Dr. Quinn. Maybe this won't finish the illustrious Quinns. But they will be mortally wounded. That's what I call checkmate.

The sudden sound of the blowers circulating fresh air through the empty laboratory broke the deadly silence.

For some strange reason it startled Dutton.

He watched the exhaust fans whisk the conveyors clean. The air tugged at the two tiny piles of ash at the edge of the disintegration chamber, then lifted and intermingled them until they swirled up and out as one.

Chapter 49

Mother and daughter perched at the edge of the massive exhaust chute. The sudden loud noise of the fans blowing ashes muffled all the other sounds around them. Zoe's shaking hand reached into a pile of rocks. She picked one up and threw it down into the opening of the chute.

Nothing! No returning sound!

The bright moonlight surrounded them, but when she stared down into the void below and tried to pierce the darkness to see something, *anything*, there was only a black hole leading down into the unknown.

And that was their only way out.

Zoe pulled Laya onto her lap. They would have to jump together into this unknown abyss. And they had to do it now. Adrenalin pumped through her body; her heart fought its way out of her chest, and at the same time her legs became paralyzed. This could be their last moment together…their last moment of life.

She had to be stronger. For Laya. For herself.

Two people were dead, not only so she and her daughter could live, but as a protest against the Corporits and their ruthless system. She and Laya had to make it, or die trying. It was the only way they could repay Nathan and Seka for their sacrifice. They would not be taken. She could not let Emory Dutton win.

Zoe looked at Laya. Her face glowed in the moonlight. She was alive, vital, so beautiful.

Zoe wanted so much for her. Wanted her to live, have a life, a real life. And she wanted to be there, too. The two of them had lost so much time; there was so much to tell her…so much she wanted her to know.

The disintegration chamber door banged open; a blast of exiting ash coated their faces, their clothes. The chute below their feet was louder now as the huge ventilation fans kicked in. The increased suction in the chute shrieked like the howl of a trapped animal that had awakened from a long sleep. The sucking air pulled at their legs.

"Where are Seka and Nathan?" Laya said, struggling to wipe her face clean of ash. When Zoe was silent, she tugged at her mother's sleeve, demanding an answer.

"They're not coming, sweetheart. They didn't make it."

Her daughter's eyes grew large, filled with tears. "Oh, Mommy!"

The lab was alive with swarming CAPOs. Their thumping boots, angry shouts grew louder. Zoe saw them getting closer as they rushed toward the open disintegration chamber.

"They're almost here, Mommy!"

A blast of static cut through the commotion. Emory Dutton's voice bellowed over the telespeaker:

"Get that woman! Get the child! Now! Don't let them get away! Get them!"

Zoe clutched her trembling daughter and stared down into the roaring blackness below.

One of the CAPOs was crawling through the inactivated disintegration chamber. His boots slapped against the wall. He was so close, Zoe could see his searching eyes behind his gas mask.

Closer, closer, he only had to reach out. "I'll get them," the CAPO shouted.

With Laya on her lap, Zoe pushed off and they dropped into the void.

Blasting air tore at her hair, pulled at her ears. They fell down, straight down; both of them shrieked in terror as darkness swallowed them.

A sudden bump jolted Laya out of Zoe's arms. Horror clawed at her chest. Her daughter was gone.

"Laya! Laya!"

Zoe's heart burst as she was spit out into a mound of ashes that billowed around her like a huge cloud. She sank down. Everything closed in, buried her.

She held her breath, pushed at the ashes above and around

her until her face was free. She coughed, coughed again, coughed harder to clear her nose, her throat of the flying ash. She flung her arms out like a drowning swimmer, trying to push through the shifting piles of snow-like powder. But she kept sinking deeper and deeper with every stroke.

"Mommy," a weak voice called out.

"Laya!"

Zoe flung herself outward, pushed forward, hand over hand toward the voice. The moonlight highlighted a limp hand poking out of the ashes. She grabbed onto Laya, yanked, yanked again, harder.

Zoe's feet landed on a solid ledge. She pulled, dragged her daughter until they broke free of the human silt. She wiped and blew the white powder from Laya's face. Her daughter didn't move, didn't breathe.

Zoe covered Laya's mouth with her own, forced air inside, breath after breath, until finally, like a puppet coming to life, Laya sat up, wheezing, coughing, spitting out ash.

Her daughter opened her eyes.

Zoe cried out in joy, kissed Laya's head, her cheeks, her neck, then started all over again with her forehead. She couldn't stop. "I thought I'd lost you forever."

Laya gave Zoe a weak smile, then threw her arms around her mother's neck.

"Look!" Zoe said, laughing, tears gushing down her cheeks at the same time. She pointed at The Organ Harvest building, high on a hill above them "We're in the clear, Laya. We're safe."

The chute had carried them far beyond the huge building complex, dumping them into a deep ravine, leaving San Francorp behind.

The End

Acknowledgements

The Group: Margaret (Peggy) Lucke, Shelley Singer, Nicola Trwst, Judith Yamamoto, and, above all, J. J. Lamb, who is always there for me, through the good, the bad, and the ugly and still loves me. Hard to believe.

Web and cover design guru, Sue Trowbridge.

Many thanks to Marcia Muller and Bill Pronzini, MWA Grand Masters and especially grand, supportive friends; to our other supportive writer-friends: Rita Lakin, Shelley Singer, Margaret and Charlie Lucke, Jaki Girdner, Greg Booi, Ellen Kirschman, Ken Gwin, Tree Gee, Julie Smith, Barbara Yeninas And to our loyal reader-friends Regina and Bill Thomas, Patti Harais, Tris Donlevy,

To my medical pals, Gabe Farkas, Katie Velick, Betty Hannigan, Sydney Yamashita—for all the medical conversations that tickled my brain cells over many years.

So many others—friends, readers, too many to mention, but you know who you are. Please believe I'm grateful to every one of you.

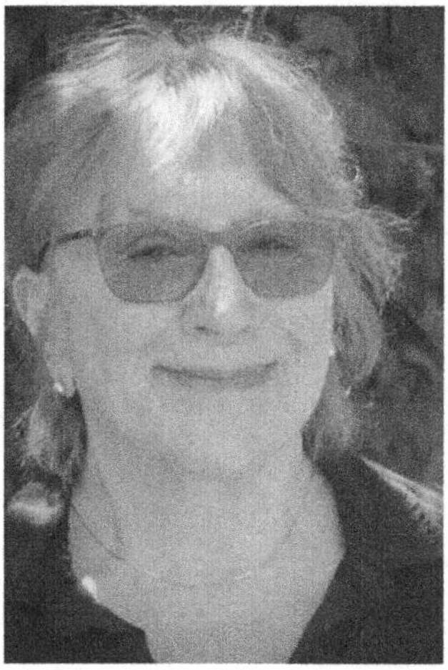

About the Author

Bette Golden Lamb, unmistakably from The Bronx, can usually be found at her desk writing, or in her studio playing with clay, or in her garden tending to some 50 rose bushes. There are times, though, when she sets all of this aside and sneaks off to the movies.

An RN, she is the author or co-author of almost a dozen novels, mostly medical thrillers, with a smattering of near-future and suspense-adventure books thrown in for good measure. Her most recent near-future medical novel is *The Organ Harvesters - Book II.*

She is also a professional ceramist, sculptor, and artist, whose award-winning creations appear in regional, national and international shows and exhibitions, and are shown in galleries.

Born in New York, her peripatetic career has taken her to live in Virginia, New Mexico, California, back to New York, Nevada, and back to Northern California, where she now lives with her co-author husband, J. J. Lamb.

Made in the USA
Monee, IL
04 November 2026

67380489R00184